Quantum Self Healing

The Power of Mandalas

Nicky Hamid

Quantum Self Healing

Dedication

This book is dedicated to my beloved wife, and life partner, Glynne who watched me go to death's door and whose compassion allowed me to freely follow my own journey rather than react to her fears for my safety. You show me the courage of a true Mother Star.

Table of Contents

Introduction: The Challenge

If you are just going to read this book and not put into practice immediately at least a little of what it is pointing to, then I strongly advise you not to waste your time. Reading just for entertainment, while feeding your mind, just digs you further into the grave of your own complacency and inertia. When you agree with an idea, a theory, or the possible validity of someone else's experience, it may help you to feel you are "right" or "on the right track", but it cannot give you the experience of knowing which your own feelings from actions will do. The New Reality that has arrived through the 2012 galactic portal is all about experience. Experiencing through your own choices. Experience that can only come about by you choosing, in any given moment, what you will allow yourself to experience, what potential you are open to, how much trust you hold in your own process and, the infinite possibilities in the unknown opportunity for each moment. It is based in your knowing of the perfected and perfecting unfoldment of a benevolent and totally connected, unified and integrated Universe that you are intimately a part of.

So if you have chosen this book because in some way you really want to experience the power of your own healing process and catch an amazing glimpse of the infinite unfolding reality of the core, the centre of who you are, you have to try the transformation process suggested. If you judge it without experiencing it then it will be a pity, because you will have missed an amazing opportunity to experience the grace, the beauty, the power of your own creative, transforming, and healing potential.

If you procrastinate and say "I would really like to try this but I will leave it until I have more time" then I ask you "how committed are you to your own well being?" If you resonate with the content of this book and see the efficacy of the transformation modality it outlines, why are you holding back? How much are you willing to trust yourself? Do you really believe that any person can heal themselves or are the growing instances of miraculous recoveries just random occurrences without causal connection to the feelings and intent of the recipient? How much do you believe in the connection between, mind, body, emotion, and spirit and the power of the cells to provide complete immunity and health recovery?

Your commitment to these and other related aspects of your reality will be tested if you put into practice, just a little of the code activation process outlined in this book. I encourage you then, to be open and, in following your own guidance, of course, do try the method without undue effort and with the expectation that, it will be very familiar to you and that you have experienced its power in another time, as a child, but you have forgotten. Enlightenment is about remembering and knowing within your being, and with complete confidence, in the goodness and holiness of You and therefore of All That Is.

If you are looking for proof that the method outlined by me works you will not find it in this book. You will find it in the reality of your experience, through your heart knowing, and through giving it a fair and playful trial.

I DARE YOU.

.

CHAPTER 1   THE NEW ENERGY

We are on the threshold of an entirely new life. The pressure of the ages is upon every human being to enter into an expanded consciousness that is available right now and that is a prerequisite for being able to maintain themselves within the energy frequencies that are the new Nova Earth.

We are just moving into the Age of Aquarius, the age of the water carrier, and for the next 2500 years the whole of life on Earth will have made a full turn, a Shift into a dynamic interplay of her physical nature with the Cosmic light waves eminating from the Great Central Sun at the centre of the Milky Way, the Source of All That Is in our galaxy.   No longer is Earth to be an isolated outpost buffeted by outside and uninvited guests. She has already made her full turn and is facing squarely her new direction in her return Home to her full and unique place in the great Plan and her conscious part in it. A plan that includes her human emissaries who will take her accumulated knowledge and share it with countless life forms in others stars systems and planets in another timeline. Human Masters with the fullness of experience of having gone into the deepest darkness, into extreme density, into total shadow, total ignorance, total distrust and hate of creation and self, fear, pain and the fullest loneliness of separation, and who are piercing through it all, with and of their own freewill. Human Masters who will share what it is like to be totally in love with All That Is, free and connected, and will know all the many ways of how to make the Shift from forgetfulness to expanded consciousness, no matter how 'lost' a consciousness may appear to be.

An entirely New Energy has been entering the very fabric of our world and us, since the Harmonic Convergence of 1987. It is now well and truly present and ever present. It flows as a great stream through every particle and atom of all that you see and sense, and all that you are. You are continually being bombarded with photons (light particles) as our solar system moves further into the photon waves from the centre of our galaxy and our sun is pulsing out increased energetic waves throughout our solar system. Every particle of matter, every pebble, every grain of sand, every rock, plant, creature and human being is receiving, in full measure, these light waves and your light quotient is increasing, your DNA field is changing and your consciousness must change to align with its expanding potential. When DNA is burst open a massive amount of light is emitted. Each DNA molecule captures countless photons and it is these that are the basis for healing and regeneration. Thus the implication of these changes for an evolutionary leap in physical development is extraordinary.

Similarly the magnetic field of the Earth is fluctuating and increasingly being fired by solar flares from our Sun. Your own magnetic field is affected likewise and you are feeling it with an increased sensitivity to the sun and in your experience of unprovoked, and unpredictable emotional fluctuation waves. You see these effects in the people around you with brief bouts of elation, longer periods of depression, and short lived emotional outbursts.

You have no option but to ride these waves of change for you made your choice by being here on Earth at this time.

The New Crystaline Energy of the Water Carrier

You are here stepping into the Age of Aquarius, carrying a physical body of water, and being constantly infused with increasing light particles which are enlivening and reviving all the reality, all the truth, and all your memory of being connected, being Unified with the Source of all life, and truly knowing the Divine being that you are.

Aquarious- The Water Carrier

Yes, and you are a water carrier. Your physical body is between 70-80% water and there is no physical animate life without water. The Divine spark of your loving consciousness has imprinted in the water a sequence for your physical development. It is the water structure which creates the double helix and the proteins without which our bodies would not work. Every seed, every embryo begins its life in water. Water gives life and has its original vitality but how you handle it, whether you bless it or abuse it, determines its quality and its effect on your body.

Water assimilates the vibrations of that which it comes in contact with and information about specific biological and energetic features. Just through your thinking and drinking you can effect the structures in water and you can change the health of your body.

Holy water, blessed water, water given loving intention all have a geometric snowflake-like structure, and the intentions that have the greatest effect on water are those that combine love and gratitude.

Water, the very nature of our planet and ourselves, and it is in water that we have the clues to our relationship with the new energy within us.

Water is made up of hydrogen (the number 1) and oxygen (the number 8). Source, is given as the One and all springing from this Source as infinite potential, and Infinity represented by the 'figure of 8", the expansion into everything manifest or made possible. And thus the uniting of these two elements, hydrogen and oxygen, two colourless, odourless gases leads to this magical crystaline substance which is something totally transparent, clear, and fluous. It has density but is not dense. And it is the basis of all organic life.

The qualities of water are so profound that it has been said that its qualities point the way to the experience of Oneness and connection to All That Is. Water is receptive and accommodating. It fits in with whatever it is in the presence of. It is soft and vital, and its absence leads physically to the hard, dry, and lifeless. It is powerful and can dissolve mountains and wash away the largest of obstacles and yet is effortless in its relentless flow. It is yielding and moves with ease and grace. It can fill any receptacle but can store within it any information copied from what it touches or is proximate to. In its clarity and stillness it reflects what is there (the truth). And in its flexibily and softness it points to absence of mind and the receptivity of feminine consciousness.

And if you are to know the Way to live in the New Energies you would do well to know the truth about the water that you hold dominion over. Carry and treat it well and drink heartedly.

We are all truly moving into a fluid state of being our body composition and the nature of the

New Energies will guarantee that. It behoves us to step into the flow of ourselves.

The Aquarian Being

What is it about the Aquarian human being that is so different and that will mark our transition? What is it that will give us the vision, strength, and courage to step from the Old cause/effect Reality of hate and suspicion, fear and pain, struggle, survival, lack, and victimhood, into one of total love, peace, harmony, self-empowerment, creativity, joy, and unity consciouness?

Freedom

The Aquarian spirit is first and foremost about freedom. Freedom of self expression, freedom of choice, freedom to explore new ideas and experiences, freedom to love, and to share, freedom to set up new adventures and to build, freedom to grow and to embrace whatever one chooses, and above all freedom to trust self and all creation, and in that freedom comes the expanding capacity for Divine eternal and total loving consciousness. Such freedom is the very basis of being human and being God as One. It was the mistrust of this freedom that seeded all the woes of the Old Reality. It was the mistrust of self and then mistrust of others that set in motion all the hurt and cruelty. And now it is the Aquarian who will take back their freedom unperturbed by the fear of others. It will be freedom that will move us all from separation to connectedness (wholeness and Oneness).

We see it in the rise of the Indigo human. The Old World shudders at the youth's apparent disregard for the law and rules of society. Yet if you examine carefully, without judgement, you will see their perceptiveness and utter contempt for hypocracy of any kind. They see through lies and deception, hidden agendas and manipulation, and though they may pay some lip service, they are not taken in and will either speak their mind or totally ignore the source and thereby communicate clearly their lack of acceptance. The Indigos are naturally telepathic so you cannot lie to them. They see through falseness though they may not have yet found their place or full voice. Even as children they have not been "hoodwinked" by the emptiness and false promises of the education system they have been forced to endure.

Knowing

It is the essence of the Aquarian human to express their freedom in exploration of their truth through experience. No longer seeking truth through beliefs that separate, or by defining of their reality through the truth of others, or some ultimate truth. Truth for the Aquarian is based on how their experience feels in relation to their own witnessing of the expansion of Source within their own consciousness and their version of reality that they explore and share. There will no longer be any need to view anything as right or wrong for humans will blossom as authentic sovereign beings who will regather their knowing of All That Is and be quietly, but quite resolutely determined about their expansion of that knowing by the infinite exploration of experience through their own unique "eyes".

Thus there will be no more futile search for The Truth but a continuing flow from one chosen experience to the next, guided by the joy of the experiencing. It will be in Now time, knowing the past or future will hardly figure.

Unity

And because of this full realisation of freedom to explore one's unique experience of reality and the many worlds and timelines that are opening up, there will be an absolute allowance and acknowledgment that other beings are also authentic sovereign beings, each with their own "eyes" and points of viewing. Each being the "Eye of God" seeing reality with the vantage point of Self but all contributing to the One All Seeing Eye, the eye of Wholeness of All That Is.

There will be no more conflict between people because beliefs, as we are seeing, are breaking down. All beliefs that separate and define "right" and "wrong" in any and all spheres of life are coming under personal and collective scrutiny and will dissolve. They will dissolve through the total removal of our decaying time sense because beliefs take memories of the past and project into the future, rules of being, rules of seeing, and rules of conduct. They say that not only "I think this way" but that "you have to think in a similar way in order for us to be in harmony". They say that the future can only be successfully negotiated with a "plan" and that if I have the "right" plan, I will be successful. But haven't you noticed how difficult it is now to make plans? The New Energies of flow we are now experiencing require us to let go and trust nature and ourselves, rather than prempt or contrive what is to come based on fear and the selective memory of past experience.

And in order to trust ourselves we are being required not only to trust Nature (the Earth), but to trust others, and this means to allow them to see differently. Seeing someone else's point of view is not necessarily adopting it, but as 'doers' it requires that we understanding it. This is part of the compassion required for the growth of our entire collective (Unity Consciousness), the capacity to "walk a mile in another's shoes". In short the 'new human' will be one who lives in a reality that is unconditional.

The Waves of Change

There are two great waves of change moving through the Universe and through the Earth and through you. These waves exist simultaneously in the same space and are in perfect harmony, resonance and synchronisation. They are setting in motion an evolutionary transformation, together moving everything to a higher vibration, a higher consciousness. Remember our connection to All That Is, and so whatever is in the large is in the small, the energetic expression of the Galaxy is seen in the smallest particle, what the Earth experiences we also experience. As above so below, as within so without.

One wave is moving outwards from an infinity point in all things, like the ripples in a pond. Initiated from a point and expanding out in all directions as great circles of change, spreading greater light, knowledge, wisdom and above all love. Its expansion opens gateways and portals to expanded consciousness and an entirely new evolutionary unfoldment. This wave is shifting mass consciousness from a third dimensional consciousness through a fourth to a fifth dimensional perspective and potential for conscious experience. It is aligning, or rather realigning, all humankind on Earth to an entirely conscious participation with All That Is. This wave provides us with new perspectives and therefore new potentialities and choices that have not been available to us previously.

This first wave makes possible the unlocking of all that has been buried within us through how we have chosen to handle the experience we have gained over numerous lifetimes. It opens the door for the second wave of the new energy from the greater infinity "outside" ourselves to penetrate within and release all the energy that has been stuck in our third dimensional consciousness. This second wave frees all the memories, all the blockages, all the experiences, and all our talents, abilities and wisdom. It makes them fully available as potentials to be made manifest by our love, intentions and choices. A theme of this second wave is to create harmony, to restore total balance in all levels and spheres of our consciousness. To align everything with the pure Divine light that you are. Thus everything that is not aligned with the truth of who you are is being currently dislodged, disengaged, destabilised, disabled, dissolved and cleared away into the nothingness from which it came. All dysfunctional patterns are being released. On every level they are being removed while simultaneously new potentialities are becoming consciously available through the first wave initiated from within you.

And so you, as a consciousness vessel, a "Holy Grail" chalice, are simultaneously being emptied and filled. Emptied by the light of creation without and filled by the light of you within. These two waves of transformation are allowing you to reconfigure yourself from the inside to the outer (physical), to remember who you really are, to reconnect with all things, to be rewired and realigned to the fullest potential of the truth of you, why you came here, and what you really want to experience and accomplish.

Thus these times are all about change. You asked for it. You cannot stop the second wave. It will open cracks in the walls of protection, of false safety and security. It will expose the caverns of emptiness, loneliness and unlovedness in your experience of yourself. It will make conscious all the unkind lies you have told yourself of who you are. It will lay bear the false identity you have clung to. All these cracks will spill out the false and will be filled by this first wave of new light that springs from your inner core at One with all Creation. You will gradually, stealthily, willingly and magnificently allow your all to be filled with the liquid light of the Source of your own being.

This second wave is a tonal wave, a wave of being that is unfolding the truth of who you are effortlessly.

The One "Rule"

In this Shift the basic rule of life has not changed. We are simply becoming more ready to own the truth of it and take charge of our own power as creators. The "Rule" is Love. Love is the life force of this and every other universe. Love is God, Goddess, and All That Is. Lover is Source. Love is the matrix that connects us all. Love is chi, the life force of connection. It is Unity and Oneness, and it leads to expansion and creating.

This love will heal the planet, transform your lives. It will open your heart and awaken your mind because it is both of these. It will move you beyond imagination and into a potential future of your highest and most Divine potential.

Implicit in the Old Rule of life is a duality consciousness, as we have known it, and spiritual growth has been hard work, discipline and detachment (separating self from the mundane). The New 'Rule' for negotiating the New Energies of transformation and expansion, is sought after and achieved by the soul, and is simply an alignment with Divine Flow, which is effortless. Therefore if your work, your life, is causing you difficulties, then you are executing your efforts primarily from your personal and ego self. In learning to live from the energy and alignment of your own soul you will live as one who is fully blended with your own soul, and your life will take on a divine elegance and ease that will allow you to do more, love more, accomplish more, feel your peace and connectedness more, heal more, receive more, and grow more.

The operational basis of life has changed and humanity is on the greatest adventure of its entire existence right now. You are a light bearer who is not only transforming naturally but has the ability to help this change be the evolutionary step that it is meant to be. Even Mother Earth and our whole solar system is moving into the unknown, and you are being given an invitation to join the journey and cocreate.

In fact, from the beginning of creation and the first moment in time, there has been only one rule and that is Love.

So transformation and healing are already a given in the life that is all around you and within you. There is nothing that you **must** accomplish to effect the changes and the healing, it is a given in this Now reality. Purely and simply find ways that from moment to moment take you into love, into your Heartspace and allow nature, your deep inner truth, to do its work and permeate all that you feel about yourself, all you are, all that you do.

Thus it is just like standing in the eye of a great circle and allowing the circle to spin and expand, transforming all events, all causes and effects, all dimensions, all moments into a new, unknown unexpected, and exciting arrangement of possible experiences. Love, trust, and allow. Go and have fun.

CHAPTER 2   INTO THE EYE OF THE SPIRAL

Little did I know that in deciding to write this book that it would lead to a deep and transforming journey for myself. It hardly occurred to me that the simple, and apparently straight forward intent to share a vision of healing and self empowerment through writing would lead to an extraordinary personal journey of healing, empowerment and liberation for me.

I had just completed my book "All You Can Be: Empowering Awakening Angels", it was mid June of 2009 and I had received my first proof copies from the publisher. While waiting for the publication process to run its course I had been imagining, creating, and writing notes, in skeleton form, for another book which seemed to be focussed on outlining a creative journey process based on the number 8 and the infinite way.

I was enthused and excited. The process of writing my latest book was a joyful and easy experience. It had taken almost exactly four months to write. Each morning I would be awake around 3.30am and write for a couple of hours. During that time the entire room was filled with a brilliant golden light and not only were my friends and guides standing with me but also, from time to time, it was very much like Waterloo Station, with light body visitors coming and going in all directions, some with such curiosity that they would peer right over my shoulder, to see what I was typing.

As I wrote the feeling of loving Presence was always there and in a very real sense, although the words I wrote came from me, it was so effortless that I have continued to feel that the book actually was not written by me, but rather it was "We" who wrote it.

Confidently I have realised that, "All You Can Be" is a book that has an energy of its own carried within the words. Because of the way it was birthed, now, not only do those who read it pick up on the Presence it engenders, but also each person who reads it contributes their own resonating Presence to the truth power of the book. A reader thus taps into, not just what is written, but the entire truth value and empowerment tone from all other readers combined. This was my original intention for the book, and it is leading to powerful transformations for readers. The intentions, words, and the feelings they provoke, have taken on a life of their own, so to speak.

Thus you can understand how I was so looking forward to repeating and expanding this experience with another book.

The Vision

It was almost 35 years ago, to the day of writing this, that I received the vision of promise of the self healing method I am about to outline. It was a time when I had been meditating every day for over a year and I was experiencing parallel worlds. Frequently I would be walking in the streets where I lived and be meeting people walking passed dressed in robe-like garments, all beaming with radiant smiles. There would be an overlay of other more futuristic buildings and a definite experience of another, yet very familiar world, that was simultaneously present. It was a mystical and consciousness expanding time for me.

One day after meditating I was sitting in the pervading peace when I became aware that I was sitting by a stream. I was in a place of great beauty, brilliantly illuminated and coloured. It was in another time and place in the Universe, since a quarter of the western sky was filled with a great blue planet and traversing it was a smaller pink moon or planet. The sky was full of yellows, pinks and blues, like a pastel coloured version of our earth sunsets.

I was a boy of about 8-10 years old and in the distance I could see my home and feel the happy presence of others who were my immediate family.

I sat by the stream I holding in my hands a large book. It was full of glossy pages. There were no words but as I turned the pages there was a large coloured circle (or disk) on each right hand page. There were hundreds of pages and on each the circle was brilliantly coloured and began to spin as soon as I looked at it. For most disks the colours on circle were painted and blended together as a series of concentric rings and resembled multi coloured CDs. Some circles were extremely intricate and some were very simple in their design and the variety of colours and patterns.

It appeared that this was my 'homework' book and before going to classes where, as children we would share our experiences, we first must have the experience. The amazing thing about this book, and the disks, or colour wheels, was that as soon as I looked at a page with any intended focus I would immediately and totally be transported into other dimensions of conscious experience, alternative realities. Looking into a coloured disk I instantaneously arrived in another dimension of time and space.

The first page I selected took me right into the stream. I became the water of the stream and could not only see back at myself as a boy sitting on the bank but I could feel the coolness and joy of bubbling and flowing across the rocks and through the reeds and grass as I flowed on.

I chose another page and I was immediately in another world on another planet. I could see and feel with all my senses the unfamiliar flora and fauna and travel anywhere at will. On other pages, if I had some discomfort or some physical ailment, just by looking at the appropriate colour wheel, I would immediately begin to move into ease and balance (heal), and the bodily symptoms would just fade away with ease. On other pages, if I wanted to taste, smell, touch or sense in any way, the key to the experience was given in the book and through a specific colour wheel. By merely looking at the 2 dimensional image on a page it would immediately activate in me either a perceptual shift or dimensional transformation or both. I was able to perceive in different ways and from points of view beyond my bodily confines and move through wormholes in space/time reality.

The vision was so powerful, clear, and real that when I came back to my present reality I knew that I had seen a promise of things that had been and were also to come and that I had already experienced this 'elsewhere'.

The experience was so real and so profoundly natural that over the next few weeks I experimented trying to reproduce some altered state. I drew a series of concentric circle and painted them in different and varying hues and colour combinations. Some of them were hauntingly alluring but staring at them produced very little in the way of other reality for me. I did find that one colour wheel I painted did relieve the headaches I had been experiencing. But eventually the vision became a promise that was yet to bear significant fruit. I was convinced, however, that somehow these colour wheels were able to initiate other subtle and immediate consciousness change in my mental, emotional and physical state.

Exploration of Consciousness through Mandala Drawing

The experience of the colour circles deeply affected me and I began to explore further through the use of mandala drawing.

It was a few years earlier that Carl Jung, a brilliant student of Sigmund Freud, had first introduced me to mandalas when I read some of his work as a psychology undergraduate. I had had the good fortune to be taught by scholars who recognised the predominating influence of the unconscious in shaping human behaviour and so my fascination with the relationship between creativity and intuition on the one hand, and unresolved psychic energy on the other, became a strong arm of my academic, clinical, and personal investigation.

Jung was extremely open to altenative subject matter and ideas. He tended to look at human behaviour from the point of view of a person's creative attempts to find meaning and order in the integration of their internal state and the world in which they experience and express. Your dreams, for Jung, would be seen as messages from you, to you, about yourself. They are your creative, and usually very ingenious and sometimes dramatic ways of processing emotions and thoughts that are in any way inhibited, or below the level of conscious awareness.

His exploration of how we explain and express meaning, especially through symbols, included the study of religion and mysticism of numerous cultures. Amongst a number of ways to unlock this human potential he became fascinated with mandalas.

Carl Jung on Mandalas

Jung began his study of mandalas with his own experience of drawing and colouring circular shapes and designs, and noticed that they somehow corresponded to his inner situation, feelings, impressions, and thoughts. He concluded after extending his study with the circular drawings of his patients, that they were therapeutic, both to draw, then to contemplate.

He made popular the Sankrit word "**Mandala**", which has been taken to mean 'centre'. The word *mandala* actually is derived from the root *'manda'*, which means *'essence'*, to which the suffix *–'la'*, meaning *'container'*, has been added. Thus, a *mandala* is a container of essence. It contains within it an expression of infinite source of SELF.

Simply put, the mandala form is the center, a *'bindu'* or dot which is a symbol apparently free of dimensions. It points to a 'seed', 'sperm', 'drop', the most salient starting point, the eye of the spiral of creation. It is the gathering center to which the outside energies are drawn, and in the act of drawing the forces, there is an equal and opposite unfolding of its own energies as it expands from this Source to the outer limit of the circle. Thus it represents the outer and inner spaces and points to the two waves of the consciousness shift that was referred to in Chapter

1. Its action is to remove the object-subject dichotomy, and any sense of duality. In the process of the creation of a mandala, patterns and forms materialize out of a dot or centre. Other lines are drawn until they intersect, creating geometrical patterns. The circle drawn around stands for the dynamic expanded consciousness of its creator.

A mandala, therefore, is so much more than a circular coloured pattern. In its simplest form it starts with the central dot. A point that is infinitely "small", whose boundaries spiral as it is amplified into infinitely large, and at any point in that expansion it can be defined as a circle. In the drawing of a mandala we are immediately drawn into, or 'entrained', to these infinities of knowing and realization. One spiraling out in expansion from the central point and one spiraling in from the circumference.

Duality thinking, which is at the root of the human dilemma and results in all our sense of separation, is represented in all our attempts to "square the circle". To contain the circle in a box, to define it rather than contemplate and apprehend it as it is. The challenge of constructing a square with the same area as a given circle by using only a finite number of steps with compass and straight edge has been proven to be impossible. Thus I am using the expression "squaring the circle" as a metaphor for doing something logically or intuitively impossible. It is like trying to make something finite out of the infinite. Mandala content can be experienced, explored, and contemplated but cannot be defined. If you try to define the experience of expansion that your personal mandala engenders, in logic, analysis, and words, its impact on your conscious awareness is clearly felt as diminished.

Jung refers to the mandala as "the psychological expression of the totality of the self." Within everyone's psyche, to one degree or another, can be found a seed-center of the self surrounded by a chaotic mixture of issues, fears, passions and countless other psychological elements. It is the very disordered state of these elements that creates the discord and emotional imbalances from which so many of us have suffered on a regular basis. It is the source of all disease. The mandala is a template for the mind, a state of peace and order, a resolution of the chaos within. As we shall see later, mandalas also act as personal portals to transformational and expanded consciousness in unison with the energy wave from the "eye of self" out into your expanded energy field.

The effects of the world within and the world without are often indistinguishable as far as your self is concerned. Internal elements (ideas, emotions, compulsions) interact freely with external elements (news, relationships, taxes) in the interface that is your mind. Understanding this exchange helps us see more clearly how certain patterns and symbolic elements from our most ancient origins have been internalised and carried through the ages, only to be unconsciously externalized in the beauty and simplicity of the mandala.

The mandala can be considered a blueprint for the essential structure of our existence, and something about this structure is instantly recognised by us. We perceive the shapes, the patterns, the elements within the mandala, we see their relationships to each other, and within that sacred matrix we recognise our self and our place in the cosmos. It is an ancient and fundamental relationship from which we have temporarily lost connection. The mandala thus becomes a key that can help us return to our centered state of being.

It is evident that the mandala is a link, though a mysterious one, between our modern consciousness and our most ancient origins. Somewhere in the vast, forgotten reaches of time lies the answer to this wondrous mystery. It is for each one of us to rediscover, and to cherish the self that has been separated. It is for us to hold the Source of energy that we are essentially one with, close in our hearts. Within it we will discover ourselves, we will find each other, and we will reconnect with the essential center of existence.

Exploration of the Effects of Mandala Drawing

I began using mandala drawing with students in my Human Potential classes at university and over the years used mandala drawing in my clinical practice, self-awareness workshops, and at spiritual retreats. Typically the person was given a paper with a large circle drawn on it and asked to draw and colour it in. Generally instructions were for the respondant's drawings to be as unrestrictive and free flowing as possible, to totally trust their first prompting. However, usually there was a little guidance given, either through directing intention towards an experience they were having or had had, or by adding some lines or design to the circle. For example, in one exercise the circle was divided into four equal quadrants and participants in turn filled each quadrant with whatever came to their awareness for their physical, emotional, mental and intuitive experience after some meditative induction was provided.

The technique was simple, enjoyable, and often resulted in insightful and self empowering answers to personal issues for participants.

When the circle was filled through a process of watching it unfold, without the person having an end result in mind, something magical was happening. Not only did participants feel considerable satisfaction from the process of colouring but often immediately or subsequently, there would be a spontaneous resolution process and a rebalancing of personal issues would result. This would occur with or without conscious understanding of what had happened. Somehow colouring a mandala initiated a change in view point that helped place the person closer to their centre and to the wisdom of understanding and/or completing something that had been unresolved.

I used mandala colouring to key workshop participants and clients into their own creative process, to free insights into their own unconscious images (eg. in dreams, visions, fears and conflict), to help them befriend their emotions, and to become more in tune with their intuitive knowledge and unlimited capacity for expansion of thought and abilty to integrate their experience.

It became very clear to me, as well as to the participants, that this drawing and colouring process was a way to express ideas and values in a different language. That this mandala language is quite natural and more dynamic, expressive and powerful than mere words, and that one of the consequences of working with mandalas was to open the mind and free the emotions in a rather unique and effortless way. It enabled a participant to see things in a different light and stimulated a diversity of thought. This in turn allowed for devising more creative solutions for day-to-day personal problems, and more generally for the creative expansion of conscious awareness. Participants became more centred, more watchful and aware, less judgemental of self, and more compassionate towards their own experiencing. In short more able to view their own internal process and external events from Heartmind.

Furthermore, those who took mandala drawing into their personal lives as a self-awareness device consistently reported to me an opening to trust in their own personal process and significant reduction in their fears. Through knowledge and the direct experience of their unconscious, they had realised that within the unconscious expression, self was a source of resolution and healing rather than being full of scary and threatening thoughts and feelings. Like a wormhole through the shadows of self. That within is an enormous power and truth, directed towards ones own greatest good and which had the potential of holding keys to many of the answers to the unfoldment of self. In a sense therefore the mandala drawing often enabled the participant to accomplish a total shift in their perspective.

Mandalas as Key Codes of Our Blueprint

It is easy to underestimate the power of a circle. History has shown that people have always sensed the healing inherent in the circular (mandala) form. It is the primal symbol of wholeness. Mandalas have been used throughout time as a tool for meditation and healing. The sacred circle can be seen everywhere we look: flowers, individual cells, our planet, galaxies, etc.

Pythagoras described geometry as 'visual music'. Music is created by applying laws of frequency and sound in certain ways. States of harmonic resonance are produced when frequencies are combined in ways that are in unison with universal law. These same laws can be applied in the creation of visual harmony. Instead of frequency and sound it is angle and shape, colour and symmetry that are combined in ways that are in unison with universal law. Geometric shapes and colour can be orchestrated in ways to produce visual symphonies that show the harmonic unification of diversity. Mandalas translate complex mathematical expressions into simple shapes and forms. They show how the basic patterns governing the evolution of life work out in most beautiful manifestation of physical form.

The circle symbolizes the womb of creation, and mandalas are geometric designs that are made through uniform divisions of the circle. The shapes that are formed from these divisions are symbols, glyphs that embody the mathematical principles, the DNA sequencing as blueprints in light encoded filaments, found throughout creation. They reveal the inner workings of nature and the inherent order of the universe.

Mandalas act as a bridge between the higher and lower realms. They are interdimensional gateways linking human consciousness to the realms of archetypes and the infinite. The relationship of light, form, movement, space and time is evoked by the mandala.

Mandalas offer a way to engage with the inherent harmony and balance of nature. They bring the principles of our unfolding nature from our luminous field into conscious awareness. They act as coded keys to our energetic blueprint. The colour codes transcend language and the rational mind. They activate the wisdom and informational sequence of the law of the unfolding of our human consciousness.

Since the new energies are growing stronger by every passing minute there has never been a more powerful time for the self activation of your own healing process. The awareness of this fact and the draw power of mandalas in this process is burgeoning worldwide. People are awakening to the profound and hypnotic attraction of geometric and circular patterns.

Though mandala drawing has been used for centuries, today just a cursory search on the internet will show that there are literally thousands of people around the world who are using the mandala forms in their work as scientists, teachers speakers, artists and healers. Indiviuals frequently share their mandala artwork in their blogs, and websites and are quite obviously using their creations as devices for transformation and healing, reporting significant improvements and changes in a variety of bodily and emotional symptoms and thought processes.

Conclusion

I therefore have concluded, from my own personal experience and research with hundreds of my students and clients, that through creating circular symbolic designs, mandalas, an increased level of self integration can develop. That this happens easily and naturally just through the process of being a participant observer in the act of drawing and colouring, and that this integration and healing occurs beyond the level of conceptual language and logical understanding. In fact preconceiving or premeditated conscious construction of pattern or images in creating the mandala will interfere and limit the extent to which new insights and resolution of imbalances within the psyche of the individual are made possible.

I have never ceased to be awed by the tremendous capacity of people to be able to experience their reality and to arrive at creative solutions in the resolution of imbalances in their life. It is so much about trusting ones own process by getting the logical processing mind out of the way of the natural and ever present internal wisdom. Literally moving from disjointed peripheral points of the mandala into the centre which includes the whole field of our subconscious and superconscious awareness for that moment in time.

In a nutshell, as soon as you begin to draw and colour within a defined circle you step into your own spiral of beingness, the universe of you. Mandala drawing can offer a profound glimpse into the galaxies or the microcosmic world of atoms, cells and particles of consciousness whirling within your being. The more allowing, accepting, open and loving you can be in that process, the more transformative the outcome will be for you. All of us are on a journey of expanding consciousness. How much more potential there has to be in an infinite universe rather than a reality bound by the definition and constriction of the logical mind and emotional victimhood. Drawing your own mandala immediately provides you with an opportunity and experience of stepping beyond duality. Of activating DNA informational sequences that unblock 'stuck' energy and unlock new energetic wave forms that activate and expand perception and the whole range of our sensing of reality.

Healing the Body

It is my expressed purpose to focus the remainder of this work on the healing of the physical body through the use of mandalas. The body is not separate from the mind, the emotions, the spirit, your consciousness "owns" them all, but we have so far looked from the wider standpoint of the power of mandalas to effect change. In the rest of the book I will primarily focus my treatment of the mandala healing process on physical body disharmony.

In the next chapter I will outline the basis of disease and the nature of self healing. We will explore the relationship between belief and healing and propose the link between colouring a mandala and the activation of the new DNA codes for healing and transmutation. Then in Chapter 4 I will provide the simplest of techniques of mandala design and execution for you to get started in your own healing activation process.

In Chapters 5 we will examine the mandala session from the point of view of developing maximum healing and growth potential. In other words, how and what you can do to enhance your session. In Chapter 6 I will outline my own rather remarkable healing journey using mandalas, and the working through of beliefs that block the power of our body to self heal.

In the final two chapters I will first outline a simple coded sequence program based on the numerical code of our DNA configuration and finally give a number of ways mandalas and healing circles can be used in your practice.

CHAPTER 3   HEALING AND DNA

I have already alluded to the possibility that drawing and colouring circles cannot only shift our consciousness into others states of being, but can also effect changes in our mental, emotional and physical health and wellbeing. We will now examine more closely what is healing and wellbeing in your physical body, how you can personally effect change at a deeper quantum level from disease and imbalance to balance and wellness. We will also begin to examine how mandala drawing can play a significant part in facilitating and enhancing the healing process.

Your Power to Heal

You have amazing power to heal yourself completely because you are much, more than just a body form. Energetically you could think of the centre line of your body (straight down your spine), as a magificent magnetic column of pure white light that is travelling up and down simultaneously. The lines of force (just like the pattern of iron filings around a bar magnet) travelling down, out the base of your spine and soles of your feet, sweeping around and up outside you in a luminous field of energy. They also travel up, out the top of your head, sweeping around and down. See them as lines of force of brilliant gold light surrounding you in a spherical cocoon of energy. This is one view of the field of you, which extends in layers up to 30 feet or more all around you. It is all you and is held through your consciousness, though you may not as yet be aware of it. A key to all the bodily transformation you desire is in the recognition and fuller identification with this multilayered, multidimensional luminous field of you.

It is not just energy, it is an information field containing not only all the potential for all you can be, but all the experiences you have ever had in all your lives, as well as all the experiences of your ancestors from your genetic lineage. The information and blueprint for anything a body has been in any lifetime of any person is available within the information field of you, the morphic field (field of the instruction set for what is possible in human form) of the collective experience of all humankind.

Health and Self Healing

All disease, bodily afflictions and pain are the result of imbalances in our energy system. All energetic imbalances are the result of interruptions in the natural and Divine flow in our consciousness field at some level. They are the result of artificial implants, or conscious restrictions we have placed on ourselves, at one time or another, and have taken on within the force field that expresses who we are, and we have at some level in our consciousness placed these restrictions in order to gain certain experiences. Through deliberately holding within our consciousness, beliefs about our separateness, our unloveableness, our limitedness, in a myriad of ways, we block the energy flow from our Source and these blocks eventually become reflected as bodily symptoms if a blockage, and its release, is not dealt with. So healing is entirely about releasing and balancing the flow of the life force within and around us.

There are numerous methods and healers that can help us to begin the release of a blocked flow and imbalance, but any effect will not last unless we ourselves remove the beliefs (the unkind lies about our powerlessness) that initiated the blocks and imbalances in the first place.

Thus it is, that in making the shift to authentic being, you are required to apply the same love to yourself that you would give to anyone else. You must take full responsibility for all that your are, all your imbalances and bring your own most compassionate point of view to bear on yourself through your love, through your forgiveness and through trusting in your own cellular community to redress the imbalances and heal completely. In doing so you give back to the whole of humankind the gift and the information of your own transformation through the contribution you make to the morphic field, because, in evolving, you add to the information available to all in the collective consciousness.

Healing and Transformation

We use the word "healing" here but it is really not the best word for what we will be doing.

"Healing" implies that there is something wrong that must be fixed. But you are a perfect expression of the One Source of All That Is. You are love incarnate, a Divine, angelic consciousness having a human experience. Everything you experience was created by you in the complete knowing of yourself and what you wanted to experience. Thus the change you seek in the bodily, emotional, or mental experience is a transformation from imbalance to balance in your energy system rather than a correction from an error. A bodily symptom is not an error. It is a signal of energetic imbalance that, once dealt with leads to wellbeing. Similarly, the emotions of anger or sadness, and the thoughts of confusion or doubt, are all sources of information about the energy flow in your body. They are a gift for your knowing and they are prodding you to make a change to a more truthful way of seeing yourself and your reality. They are reflecting in your body and impacting your conscious awareness until you take notice of what they are telling you about your off-centeredness, the inharmonious flow in your energy system. They remain in your experience until you let go of the associated belief that denies who you really are. The release of these thoughts will let flow an emotional reaction that, if allowed its expression, in love and forgiveness, will cleanse and free your energy flow.

So whenever you go to use the term "healing" try using "transformation" instead, intending the desired change to be towards free flow from a state of restricted flow. And it is here we have a great clue to healing. Anything that increases the free flow in our energy system will directly contribute to our healing. For example, increased intake of pure energised water, increase in oxygen intake through conscious breathing of the life (Light) force to afflicted body areas, increase of blood flow within the body. An easy, relaxed, playful, and less serious attitude to life i.e "going with the flow", aides in the removal of beliefs that restrict the expression of our joy, removal of attachments that bring fear of loss and are based on the lie that we need to strive to survive and, therefore, are not eternal. Anything that will help you to let go will increase the flow. Anything that will aide the flow will in turn help you to let go. Simple isn't it?

It has become a given that the New Energies are automatically and quite naturally leading us all to total wellness, they are programmed for health. Being in its flow makes available the information for a perfected body blueprint of our highest imagination and deepest longing. All that is required is for us to allow for an open flow of these energies.

DNA and a New Blueprint for Complete Wellness

The unfoldment of you, your divine spirit, the whole complete and infinite nature of who you are is made manifest through a coded light sequence of your essence. Golden light threads of infinite variety and potential expression patterned according to your Divine will at One with All That Is. This pattern of the manifestation and expression of who you are and your potential becoming is inlaid with coded informational sequences for the outpouring of the expression of you and the nature and form you have intended for your next experience. This is your Divine blueprint and we have called it 'DNA'. We can imagine it as a set of 12 matrices each with its prescribed sequence, each with their own wave form, and each with their own place in the vibratory ranges of the fuller, more complete energy that we are, in expanded consciousness. But of course it is much, much more than we could conceive in our mind or express in words for it exists in sound and light expression.

These 12 strands of DNA provide six paired coded sequences of action and expression for the evolution and involution of the full and whole manifestation of the vessels and energy forms in which, and through which, you express your Divine nature, your Presence. One pair only is needed to provide the sequence for all physicality of being as we presently know it. All 12 pairs are needed for the fullest expression of who you are as a spiritual, light being, in a physically perfected form.

It is now, in this time of the great shift in consciousness, that all the DNA is being freed of the veil of unconsciousness (and apparent randomness), and sequences for the bridge between vibrational tones (dimensions or worlds) are becoming activated by our very intentions and conscious readiness. All of humanity is being 'rewired' as the new sequences for our unfoldment and evolution take root and flourish. The influx of light energy, photons, in all physicality, requires a corresponding evolutionary transformation in the nature (vibratory rate) of the physical body. There is no stopping it for the desire of humanity for 'something more', 'something better', and 'something truer' is too great and now too much of one voice to be blocked. The collective human consciousness now expresses such an attractive force that expanded consciousness is inevitable. The call to action has fired the 'lost' or 95% 'junk' DNA into returning, and the unfoldment of the consciousness of the truth and magnificence of humankind is now well underway.

The action of the DNA and its sequence of the unfolding prescription for wholeness of being cannot be described, nor can we understand or manipulate it from any point of technology or "spiritually wise" conception. To do so is to retread the path of Atlantian times where our technological brilliance and spiritual knowledge lead to our own downfall. DNA provides, with its encodings, the prescription for the manifestation of the Law of your own Unfolding, or we could say, the Law of your own ascension.

In other words the fact, the reality of your own evolution, your own ascension, is already assured. It is written, it is encoded, you have already willed it through your love and from the fullness of your Being. It will come naturally and without any need to know consciously anything about DNA or its action. The waking up to the fullness of who you are is assured. You have decreed it to be so. How long it will take and whether the ride will be bumpy or a joyful surfing on the sea of change, is entirely up to you. It is in your own freedom that you will choose to experience the next chapter of human evolution.

So becoming well is not about speeding the process of DNA growth, nor rooting out the blocks and the impediments to its expression. It is not about knowing the ins and the outs of the levels of DNA and how they interrelate or can be enhanced or can even be short cut. There is no shortcut to ascension. The unfolding sequence of encodements from your DNA requires the full and proper balance of all levels of who you are as a most magnificent Divine expression in physicality.

This is accomplished by knowing and full acceptance of the truth that the prescriptions for your greatest good, your fullest expression and the perfection of your physical form is already in progress. Your DNA codes are being constantly 'downloaded' and the resultant effects and actions work their way through at all levels of your being to where they are appropriate. They are timed and placed to perfection.

So the whole thing is easy. There is no effort required. Effort is from the old survival mode, it comes from the fear based belief that progress requires concerted and prolonged action. Your DNA already contains all the codes, the knowledge and the perfection of plan for your greatest and optimised transformation. All you need to do is relax a little, love more fully, and really, honestly, and deeply learn to trust your own process generally and your body consciousness in particular. I am reminded of Jesus when asked about his journey saying "My yoke (my union) is easy, my burden is light (Light)."

And so you can think of your DNA as a set of coded sequences of Light, colours, patterns, sound, tastes, smells, touches and numerous other sense impressions we have yet to fully realise. These codes activate processes, and experiences that lead not only to our physical growth, harmony and balance, but also to expanded capacities of perception and knowing. The codes are already written and can be activated through simple acts of loving receptivity.

Most of these codes are not new, you have already recognised such codes in drawings, sense impressions, crop circles, patterns and mandalas, in nature in the flowers and seeds. Such perceptions leave you with strong and deep feeling of something profound and something so familiar but unable to be spoken. These codes are in a Language of Light and they are at the core of who you are. Therefore, of course you would know them. They bare an aspect of the total expression of who you are, have been, and are becoming.

Our Reality and Mandalas

Our Reality is fashioned moment by moment through the outpouring of an infinite and expanding expression of consciousness expression. It could be likened to the pattern of expanding circular waves created by a pebble dropped into still water, only it is constant and in all directions. This constant expression of self is patterned by the form and the dimension in which it is expressed. Certain patterns make up each reality expression. Thus particular templates form unique reality expression, one of which is the particular three dimensional physical reality that we share. It is a patterned matrix of Light codes (adamantine particles) and their expanded sequences. These Light codes can be represented in mathematical and geometric form.

The fabric of the world you experience, therefore, is like a perpetual pulsing of the expression of patterned codes of light and sound, and sense impression. A specific sequence leads to a specific experience, it is reflected in the pattern of the Light expression.

The power of the mandala lies in this natural eternal process of expanding circular waves of consciousness expression. The geometric codes lead to a potential of expression at all levels. As you wake up, become conscious of the greater depth of you, each manifestation of the expanding waves of the expression of you is laid bare for you to play with. So the geometric design templates become under your influence as you 'ride with them" as part of your expanded consciousness. Mandalas are so powerful because not only do they represent this process, they immediately key your consciousness into this creative and creation process of circular wave generation of reality and consciousness expression. They spark you into an, "internal" experiential process that is the very nature of who you are, The more nearly the mandala echoes the codes and patterns of your inner truth expression the more immediate and profound the simple act of viewing the mandala will be. A mandala can key you into, an experience if it matches, approximates or resonates with its original coded sequence. Simply viewing a mandala can activate experiences at any level, physical, emotional, mental, or spiritual, and the more representative the mandala is of the geometric code templates in the morphogenic field the more directly it will affect your physical body.

It appears that simply colouring in a mandala, choosing both colours and design on the basis of sensing and feeling rather than preconceived decision or preference, can be sufficient to effect bodily change. Certainly I have amassed much testimony to this fact where my clients and students have reported numerous instantaneous and long term removal of physical symptoms such as headaches, pains of all kinds both deep seated and from minor accidents, viral infections, allergies, and hypertension, to name a few. These have occurred independent of their expectations since most were drawing mandala for self awareness purposes and the physical changes for them were an additional surprise outcome.

Putting it All Together

Your body is a community of around 100 trillion cells, a community consciousness of immense potential. It knows what to do to create, regenerate , and heal. It knows how to balance and maximise all its natural functions and how to live well and fully in the environment of Earth. It knows where to go to obtain the information required to make any adaptation for its next evolutionary leap.

What it cannot do is fulfil its proper growth, maintenance and evolution if the environment, the consciousness that has initiated its formation,

you, is not listening to its wisdom. And the wisdom of body consciousness is what we have called, "instinct", and we have relegated it to 'animal' in a derogatory sense, and have harboured seeds of distrust and hate towards our own community.

So we are in the process of taking back all that we are and through illness, disease , pain and discomfort our body is asking us to look and to listen to what it has to say and how we can help provide the environment in which it can thrive and evolve. And the change is not in diet regimes, or any particular health oriented practice per se. It is in the unconditional love of self and the coming together of a total unconditional trust in our body to do what it was created to do. The fundamental move we can make then, is a change of heart. To truly listen to our body, trust the impulses we get from day to day, and develop the full respect for the knowledge and power of our body consciousness to manage its own community for us.

To do its work of transformation our body needs to discard all the irrelevant information it has gathered through generations and retrieve all the relevant information from the light (information) packets contained in the newly forming DNA, situated literally at arms length, in a lattice network of light in the extended field of our consciousness. This is a very easy and natural process if we can only allow our bodies to do it and step away from the need to "meddle" all the time as if our mental mind could comprehend the enormity, complexity and intricacy of evolutionary timing. So in fact we do not need to concern ourselves about our DNA at all, it will take care of itself. Our only concern is our consciousness and that is all about holding our own space for love. The evolution of consciousness is available to all without exception. Each of us walks in Source, for Source is the origin, the path and the destination of us all. In increasing our connection to Source and our experience of our own lovingness, DNA will change, evolve, and fulfil its expression totally and perfectly.

Our job, as it were, is to provide the environment in which our body conscious can do its work in freedom. As we free ourselves from the bonds of unlovedness, we open the doors to an environment in which body can heal quickly and thrive. When you colour a mandala this is exactly what you are doing, stepping into a state of playful openness, listening to what is calling you (your body consciousness as one source) and filling the "little universe" with light and geometric form which then activates the release of resonant information in your field such that your body can respond to the new information; 1) because it is ready for it, and 2) because you are allowing it. In the act of mandala colouring you have dropped both the need to control and the need to know what you are doing before you do it.

I ask you to think of these questions as we move on to the creating of mandalas. How well do you know and love your body consciousness? Are you embracing, trusting and accepting your body consciousness through the symptoms you are experiencing? Do you believe wholeheartedly that your body has its own conscious knowledge and power to guide you through the undoing of all the old patterns and the creation of new ones? Can you treat your body with the loving trust and care that a Master would give to every other person? Do you love your body enough to allow it to fully bring itself back to you? That it is part of you in your expanded Self? Acknowledge your body consciousness, give it your love and its freedom to develop its evolution back into your Beingness. Allow the Law of your own physical evolution to be in the hands of your body.

CHAPTER 4 HOW TO CREATE A MANDALA

The method is simplicity itself. It requires no training, healer, or therapist. Just you, a quiet space, a piece of paper with a patterned circle drawn on it, a set of coloured pens, pencils, pastels, or crayons, and, if possible, access to the internet.

The more you do it the more it will work in your life. At the very least you will become aware of subtle and not so subtle changes, in your body, your emotional tone, and a slowing down of your internal dialogue.

Activation of Your DNA Codes

Before we outline the procedure for alignment to ones DNA codes there are a number of reminders to be made. First know that it is not about initiating the process of the unfolding evolution of your new body, the new you. The whole plan for your expanded consciousness and perfected being is already underway. It was born out of your desire and intention to expand your consciousness and wake up to the conscious ownership of all that you can be through physical expression, and all that you are. The New energies have been working within you to increase your capacity to receive, hold, transmute and reflect an increased number of frequencies in your body for some years now. It is initiating the growth of dormant and new energy centres (chakras) and their crystalline receivers/transmitters, rewiring your brain, and forming the new electrical bonds that will allow for the structure of a physical body that will live freely and intentionally in the higher frequencies of a fully blended human being.

Secondly the changes that are happening, while affecting us all, are also unique to you as an individual. A quite specific and wholly integrated process is underway in which the what and how of this monumental change in your experience of yourself, has a sequence and timing that is uniquely your own.

No one has experienced exactly what you have experienced, no one can experience what you experience, and thus no one will have the identical experience of their own consciousness expansion that you will have. You have exclusive access to your own experience.

Thus I encourage you to follow your own guidance with regards to the technique that is outlined and not to be bound by rules or the old pattern of "doing it right". 'Right' will be following your own nose. It is all about trusting your own nature, Your own process, your own inner guidance, and stepping out of your mind contructions based on others opinions of who and what is "right' for you.

The expansion of the consciousness of humanity cannot be stopped. You cannot stop it within yourself even if you tried. You can make the journey very rough on yourself but you came here to expand, to connect, to blend, and succeed you will, unless by some perverse decision you choose not to.

You can however facilitate your journey by using devices that remind you to allow, that open your consciousness to inner processes, that aid in activating the energy coded sequences for the necessary rebalancing in the energetic systems of body, mind, and emotion that must occur.

Every human being on this planet was born to create, was born to express and explore, through all their faculties, their capacity to separate, magnify, and blend, energies. Creative expression in this sense is any activity whereby a person expresses themselves intentionally to change their environment vibrationally.

Every child who is given the opportunity, as soon as they have the motor skills to hold a pencil or pen, loves to scribble, draw and paint, and if you can key yourself back to that enjoyment and the freedom of yourself to express then you are already present in your healing process. You may have an underlying intention to activate through, colour and pattern, the information sequences of your DNA but this you are advised to put aside when you actually sit down to create in a mandala creating session.

Creating Your Mandalas

We will start the simplest way possible because what your session is about is enjoying a creative activity rather than engaging in some kind of self-therapy. Apart from the fact that you are intending to initiate a transformation process within the field of you, this is a session for the joy of an experience in creating something. There is nothing else that must be experienced. There is no logical or conceptual understanding that is expected to result, nothing to cling on to or hold in your mind, and there is no expectation of some blinding flash of illumination or insight. It is simply sitting quietly and enjoying watching a little universe of colour unfold before your eyes as you create it.

The mandala itself will call from your field whatever is needed into your body consciousness for your body to do its work. It is being a peaceful watcher and your enjoyment in the effortlessness of the experience, that is all that is required of you consciously.

Where to get your Mandala Drawings.

Initially it is much easier to create with a good template and guidelines, because it will allow you to be involved with the colouring rather than the drawing. In fact the method outlined here and which is the basis of all that is outlined in this book is based on predesigned circular mandalas.

The first step is to obtain mandala drawing

templates. I recommend that initially you get yours from a stock of literally hundreds of drawings and patterns available free for download on the internet. You can download free mandala templates from any of the sites given at the back of this book. If you want more just Google "mandala drawings".

You can draw your own but this is unnecessary. Later I provide simple instructions for doing this if you want to extend what is covered here.

If you don't have a computer you could get a friend to print a few for you or email me and for a small fee I will send you a file of a set of 100 mandala drawings to use as is or modify according to your own inner guidance. My contact details are at the end of the book.

In making your selection for any session it is important to have a reasonable number of mandala drawings available to choose from. Your inner guidance, (body consciousness) knows what it needs so will make the best of what ever you have available but the more mandalas you have to choose from the greater the flexibility and room for enjoyment there will be. In having many to choose from try not to make heavy weather of your decision of which one to choose for any given session, trust your first reaction.

With regards to which mandalas to include in your stock there is no hard and fast rule. Choose patterned circular mandalas to start with. Avoid using mandala drawing, with an identifiable object eg heart shape, leaf drawing, face etc. Figures and motifs that have meaning instantly put restrictions and confines on the nature of your creation through the memories and associations they provoke. You can do that another time.

Some examples of mandalas I have used are given in Figure 1 and 2 and include both simple and more complex designs. I make sure that I include in my selection a blank or concentric circles design because sometimes there is a prompt to fill the space with something entirely generated intuitively. Other times the use of sacred geometry designs (Figure 3) or even crop circles designs (Figure 4) may have a draw power (see internet downloads at the back of this book).

Have at least 50 at your disposal and either print off a whole selection or choose from your saved file and print as required after you have

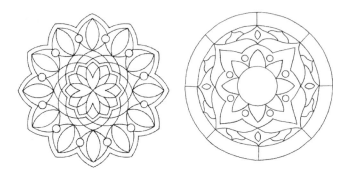

Figure 1 SIMPLE MANDALA DESIGNS

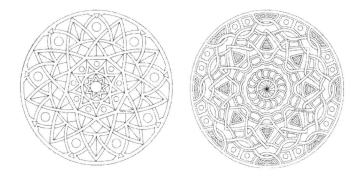

Figure 2 COMPLEX MANDALA DESIGNS

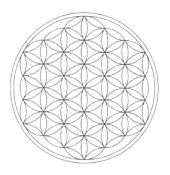

Figure 3 SACRED GEOMETRY -The Flower of Life

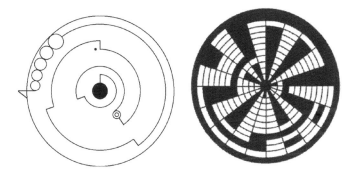

Figure 4 CROP CIRCLES

made your selection for any given session. Find a place that is relatively peaceful and where you will not be disturbed. I enjoy doing them outside on warm days. It will not disrupt the process if you are called away, because it can be resumed at any time. It is better and more satisfying to be able to continue until you are finished or ready for a break. It is just important that you don't be frustrated if you are interrupted. Just try to give yourself a place and time where you can have the maximum enjoyment of your peace.

Doing it with children or with others is fine but initially try doing them alone. Both type of sessions are beneficial but the experience is often entirely different. Again trust both yourself and circumstances, there is no hard and fast rule.

So you now have a resource of mandala drawings and you let one of the drawings choose you. You let your first reaction guide you and regardless of whether you like or dislike that particular design, your being drawn to it will determine your choice for that session.

Choosing your Colours

You can fill in the mandala design with colored pencils or markers pens (felt tips). The finer the drawing tool, the more refined your mandala will be. Crayons give a much cruder appearance than, say, Staetdler marker pens (my personal favourite and most popular to use).

Felt tips are quite sufficient just make sure you purchase a good range of colours. They are bright and clean and easy to use and give a strong striking result with the mandalas.

Oil pastels allow you to do shading while many enjoy using coloured pencils that have a lighter touch with colour. If you have confidence with a brush then paints give so much versatility and surprise.

Let a colour choose you. Whatever colour attracts you at that moment. When you have finished using it just continue with whatever next colour appeals to you in that moment. One colour on the mandala invites another, like a guest who asks to bring their friend to your party. Start colouring. Don't think about your choice of colour too much and don't worry about matching colours. Let your instincts guide you. After you've begun with the first colour, the rest will follow naturally. Avoid being biased to just colours you like.

Start colouring anywhere on the mandala, anywhere in the shapes and spaces in any order. It does not have to be orderly or even symmetrically coloured. This is totally a spontaneous process without any rules apart from the initial intention to totally endorse your energy bodies capacity to transform and for you to enjoy your creative session. Do exactly what is satisfying in the moment. Go slowly, taking in as much as you can before moving on. The mandala holds the power of unity, healing, balance, and wholeness and it will do its work without any concerted, focused effort on your part.

When you are finished try to avoid asking for others opinions or analysing them in any way. There is no right or wrong way to colour the Mandala. Be prepared to be surprised and delighted. You will usually be left feeling very content with your result. Contentment is our natural state of being.

Additional Optional Practice

None of the following is necessary for the DNA activation to occur but the following practices can certainly facilitate the process and help cement the efficacy and strength of your confidence and experience in the whole process.

Before you begin close your eyes. Breathe in through the nose, and out through your mouth, and feel your body relax, let tension go. As thoughts arise or you become aware of physical distractions, simply acknowledge them and then let them go. Do not attempt to force thoughts from your head, or feelings from your body. Accept them as part of the experience. Focus your energy into your heart until you can feel your energy flowing between your heart and your arms and hands. Keep breathing and stay still and centered until you are ready to open your eyes.

When you have finished your mandala. Gaze at your mandala with slightly unfocused eyes. Keep breathing, deeply and evenly, letting the oxygen flow in and the toxins flow out. Look deeply into the center of the mandala, trying to blink as little as possible. Don't focus on the details of the mandala, just allow yourself to notice the overall effect of it. You may be attracted to certain parts, patterns and colors. Let your thoughts come and go as you gaze. Don't look for meaning just let your consciousness absorb it totally, helping to register its imprint for internal processing. Let it imprint on your conscious awareness.

Date the mandala and put it in a folder or even better you can hang your mandala on a wall in a prominent, well lit, spot (eg. on your fridge) where you can easily view it and let it catch your eye from time to time.

Drawing your own Mandala

If you don't have a mandala drawing template, or you would prefer to draw your own mandala then here are some simple guidelines.

Draw a circle on a blank piece of A4 paper with either a compass or something round (like a bowl) as a guide. Find the centre of your mandala. On a mandala template, the centre will be marked. If drawn with a compass, the hole in the paper is the centre. If drawn with a plate, draw a light line in pencil that halves the circle from the top to bottom, and then another line from the left side to the right side, where these lines cross, and you have four equal segments, will be close to the centre.

Keep your mandala symmetrical, this will make it look nice. You will line up the motifs you use along directional lines. Think of a compass, with lines North-South, East-West, NE-SW, and SE-NW,etc.) If you have a mandala template, these will be marked on the paper. If you're drawing your own template, you'll need a ruler and protractor to mark some lines lightly on your mandala. Using 45° angles is a good standard, you will end up with 8 lines. You can just approximate the lines, but it won't work as well.

Draw a small shape in the middle of the circle with a pencil or a marker. A diamond or square, a circle, or a star, in fact any shape that presents itself to you.

Draw another shape outside this first shape. Repeat this shape in a ring all around your centre motif keeping the same position relative to the line. Keep going, drawing new motifs in expanding rings, as you work toward the outside circle of your mandala. Easy motif shapes include teardrops, fans, spirals, geometric shapes, and any other forms you like, but avoid using shapes that represent any definable object, such as butterflies, birds, dolphins, etc. Repeat some of your shapes in different sizes and introduce new ones as you go. Draw some shapes on the directional lines, and some shapes between the lines, to make a more satisfying design. This is especially important as you move outward, where there's more space between the lines.

Try overlapping some motifs; this creates new and interesting shapes, which still harmonize with what you've drawn so far. As you move outward, your motifs may be larger since you have more space to work with. You can then start putting one shape inside another, again creating more interesting shapes.

You may find yourself wanting to go back to add something to a previous ring. That's fine. It should be an entirely intuitive process. The mandala is finished when it *feels* finished to you. It can be very simple or complex. There is no rule.

If you've drawn in black pen, you may want to scan or photocopy it before colouring your mandala. That way you can colour it more than once, and share it with others to colour.

Finally you can speed up this whole process of making your own templates. First draw a circle of suitable size. Cut it out and fold it evenly three time so you have your circle divided into eight segments. Now while it is folded, with sharp sissors cut out various shapes. When you are satisfied open the circle up to reveal your mandala. You can now use it as a template to trace around on a drawn circle and then add any finishing touches you like.

This entire process of drawing your own mandala can enhance and extend your experience.

Putting a Spin on it All

It was quite clear to me early in my experimenting years ago that as soon as I had completed colouring a mandala design mostly it would appear to spin when I concentrated my gaze at it.

On gazing some report spin outwards while others experience movement towards the centre. There is frequently a definite sensation of the design spinning either towards the centre or from the centre moving outwards as if looking into a rotating vortex.

In fact this is not surprising since everything in the Universe spins. Atoms, particles, planets, stars, galaxies, even our body field. The chakras we are most familiar with are themselves energy vortices of entry and exit from our physical body. They spin, and the speed and direction of their spin is related to balance or imbalance of specific glands and organs associated with the energetic input of each chakra. Imbalance in chakra energy flow is similar to the wobble that occurs when a gyroscope or top spins at a slow speed before it comes to rest.

Perceptually we usually only see one spin direction at a time but in fact there always simultaneous spin in two direction in the same space (just as there are two waves in the New energy we saw in Chapter 1). When we look at the spokes of a spinning cartwheel, as it speeds up they spin in one direction, then they oscillate back and forth, and then settle as if they were motionless again. Remember how, with my vision in Chapter 2, the coloured discs in the book "of experiencing" appeared as circles of concentric coloured rings. This is just what you would see if you spun a coloured mandala design at a certain rate of spin.

What is now clear to me is that when completed the coloured mandala spins and the spinning arrangement initiates the DNA to form spiral threads of varying hues and lengths. These in turn vibrate, give off light, and activate cellular memories which energise growth and specific regeneration in the physical body.

After Creating a Mandala

When colouring these circles, you shift your attention from external preoccupations and concerns and connect to your own inner space. This inward attunement normally has a calming, relaxing, refreshing, and energising effect. It most definitely takes the creator into a meditative state.You will feel more centered, more calm, both during and after the session.

The simplicity and natural attraction of the mandala draws you into a private process of self-watching and self-expression for which you need no dependence on a guide or therapist or outside consultant. In the search for the trigger to the natural unfolding of your own self-transformation you can sit down anytime you want to, colour a circle, and capture a reflection of what you need next to initiate in your own process and this is accomplished through feelings rather than any thought. You are tuning into and tapping your own internal wisdom of Self. It is through the mandala that you will be able to release where your energies are blocked, and where your resistance lies, in whatever ways you are stuck. The comprehension and need to understand is put aside and may or may not come later but it will be after the change has been intitiated.

A mandala colouring session can have a profoundly integrating effect on your life. It can help you connect to, accept, love, and learn from the very center of yourself, as you are learning to live ever more freely and creatively. One of the greatest challenges in life is to discover and nourish the deep springs of inner wisdom that flow within us, and spending time with colouring mandalas encourages your inner genius to awaken, communicate, and express itself directly to awakening self. You will find that there is a very strong carry over effect on to other activities in your life.

Time with your mandalas will help you see the larger cycles that operate in your life if you do them fairly regularly and then review a series of drawings that have developed over time. Often the comparison will be profound but usually the insights, though clear, will be beyond words to describe. It will be knowledge in feeling, a knowing.

We need to find ways to connect to our inner depths, to heal our wounds, and nurture the growth of new potential within us. Mandala colouring is a most creative, direct, and transformative way to accomplish these.

It is important to reiterate that each person is changing within the Law of their own Unfolding. Thus there can be no hard and fast rule of what will happen in any given session. The effects of a session will be entirely determined by what your need is and where you are within yourself. However, people frequently report that bodily symptoms change during and after their colouring sessions. The diminishing and/or complete relief from feeling unwell or experiencing various aches and pains is commonly experienced.

Furthermore, because in the process you are

moving and freeing energy, opening up portals for your transformation, there can be energy shifts that range from mild to quite dramatic. It has not been uncommon for participants to report feelings of being totally drained, as if they have processed a great deal of emotion, or have had a long and arduous 'workout'. If this happens make sure you rest well, don't try to analyse it. It can be quite understandable since you will have released 'stuck' energy. Energy that has taken a great effort for you to maintain the block you were carrying. Of course you will now be tired because you have allowed the truth of its release to be present and now there needs to be a time for recuperation.

On the other hand, at other times you can feel rejuvenated and invigorated after your session, whereby the energy, or chi (life force) that you have 'given away' has returned to you.

Mandala colouring can lead to the same "miraculous", results for any disease or affliction and I will discuss this later in Chapter 6 in detail.

Finally, BEWARE mandala colouring is highly addictive and there is no known cure. It will open portals to your soul and to the great unknown within you. It will initiate change that is natural, subtle, and profound. It will lead you into expanded perception of yourself and the reality that is opening up before you. Life will become more unpredictable, less compartmentalised, more fluid and joyful.

In a nutshell, colouring a mandala will CENTRE you. It will bring you to the place of Heart where all things are possible in your evolving. It is just like coming HOME, and it is ineffable.

CHAPTER 5   OPERATION OPEN HEART: GET OUT OF YOUR OWN WAY

The opimal state of healing is to have absolute trust in yourself. Trust that whatever you are doing will lead to greater good. The moment you can be in the place of complete trust in yourself and your own process, transformation happens, healing happens, growth happens, evolution happens, your greatest good happens. You are creating your own life and you are no longer concerned with trying to control the outcome, you are learning to get out of the way through dropping your mind, surrendering to a higher inner knowing, and owning the knowing of total benevolence. No doubt, no analysis. The knowing that everything is created by you for your highest good, greatest expansion, and fullest joy and clarity of life. Trusting your body, when you are sick, to find its way through with ease, no matter what it feels like. You created it for the love of self. When you can truly say to yourself "I created this", you stop sweating the small stuff and worrying about what is going to happen next and it opens up all the possibilities of the "sickness" to the unblocking, the rebalancing, the recalibrating for your highest good, including the perfection and harmony of your body experience. Then the symptoms of the imbalances can resolve and dissolve. You can move into the flow of this state quite easily and naturally when you colour a mandala.

And it may initially take faith, but not faith that is blind in that it hopes for rescue and does not know. It is a faith that is finding the "feeling good about" feeling, without the evidence that backs up the healed change immediately. It is an expectation and an owned Presence of wellbeing. The change is in a learning to ignore the reality of the past that has had your undivided attention, that has kept you hypnotised, in shock, in sleepiness, and just for a little time putting it aside and diving into creative expansive expression. And if you do this your reality will do a flip, a quantum leap.

As soon as you decide to take a mandala and colour it in you enter your "healing session". In that moment you are implicitly choosing the space between doing and being. From choosing a mandala pattern to the completion of colouring you are in the place where transformational energy is initiated. It is a space where you are allowing higher self, higher purpose, to have freedom through your permission, to express its natural flow through your cellular form, and emotional/mental field.

Your willingness to enter the state of play and enjoyment, without the massive thought projections you normally fill your conscious awareness with, provides the space in which a healing transformation will naturally take place.

Furthermore, when done the activation, being initiated by your playful invitation through action, will have sparked a synchronous resonant chain reaction informational light sequence, uniquely appropriate for you, to begin the reprogramming of cellular memory and the rebalancing of your bodily system, releasing emotional/mental blocks.

The processes are made permanently active and the resultant balance in your energy system is continuous. Any bodily symptom may take just a few hours or many days to disappear, and as there are often layers to many of the blocks to ourselves, sometimes a number of sessions could be required for complete transformation.

From Stillness to Oneness

Stillness is about non-definition, about no-thing. If you perceive an object that has been given definition in your world, you can go to the heart of it to find no-thing. Going into your own heart space you have the ability to take away the definition from any object and then you allow it to release itself to you again. Every object that you see around you wants to merge its energy with you because it belongs with you.

Material objects, like your chair, your clothes, your jewellery, the house or the car, do not desire the separation that you give them. You have been taught to separate your reality from yourself. Every object around you, however, wants to unify again with you. It loves you. This does not mean that all of a sudden you will see the closet come towards you and go back inside of you. The closet can still be a closet, the chair remains chair, and a person can still be a person. It simply wants to blend with you, as it is you. Blending does not mean their form stops; it means being one and recognizing that oneness once again. The singularity of unified stardust if you will.

It is all about the intent. In the no-thingness you allow the I AM inside of you to reintegrate the things that you see around you. In doing so, you allow the I AM its breath, its existence. It is always present, but when you allow it to flow from you into all things, you merge together as the heart of all things and you become the breath of Awareness. In entering your mandala , if you allow it, this is what happens.

Every molecule, every bit of matter, be it around you or inside of you, consists solely of three things: **light** which creates **color**. Together they create a **sound**: the singing of the **DNA**. The DNA in your field begins to unwind and release light, the information light packets. Some would say it is sound that is creating the light, but the truth is that the order really doesn't matter. The order doesn't even exist because it is an infinite concept to begin with and it can't be classified in a linear way. Sound and light are in fact one and they are creating each other as you are choosing your reality into existence.

It would be wrong to say that the light, colour and song within all things is similar to yours. It isn't similar at all, it **is** yours. It is yours to emit and to create with. It is redundant to separate you from 'You' and it is time to take back this divine, creational power of the One source that you are, as a shared consciousness.

You have forgotten this truth by the illusion of separation that a duality point of view creates, so that you could not see the light in all things and even if you were to see it, you wouldn't recognize it as your own. Thus you became distracted and could not recognize the power of your body to heal because you lost the belief in your own sovereignty. What happened was definitely not a natural process. You were made to believe that you were small and separate, while you are all-powerful and an expression of oneness. Recognizing this, is taking up your power. It is true love.

When you understand that your teacher/leader and you are the same, you will never give your power away again. When you understand that your body knowing and you are the same you will never again give your power of transformation (healing) away.

Instead of following the leader in your

mandala session you are choosing to follow Self. Following the Self incorporates recognition of the I AM in you and in all things around you, and all that is around you is built up from the light-colour-song that you are.

Letting Go in Simplicity

I could have written this book in a couple of sentences. I could have written it all as "Simply grab yourself a mandala pattern drawing and an array of colours. Sit down and allow yourself the total freedom to enjoy colouring the whole thing in. The most benevolent transformation of you will be facilitated". That is it, done. But this is not enough for most minds. The mental mind wants reasons, wants to be convinced and even when convinced it will find reason why you should doubt your own power, the power of your heart. It will never stop, it will always want it to be more complex than it is. The "little' mind is not happy with the fact that transformation is through the language of light which it cannot grasp. It will not allow it to be so simple after all your struggle. You are going to have to speak strongly and lovingly to it, that it must step aside with regards to any control of the changes you are initiating.

Things heal because you allow them to heal.

There is no such thing as an accident. What you think are accidents, a car crash for example, really happen because you are attempting to move energy out, even though it may be experienced as extremely painful. The shock of the incident gets you out of your brain because of the pain, you can't even think. When this happens there is a tremendous infusion of your Divine energy, Yourself.

You get the immediate release of things that no longer serve you. You may have been trying to get rid of the energy by emotions, by mind (gone for therapy). The injury is not a mistake it is a way of release and infusion (healing) and a broken limb could be better than it has ever been if we have allowed the process.

Healing is very quick combined with new energy. There is really nothing wrong with you unless you like playing that game of being sick. You are acting being a human, you are acting as someone having physical problems, etc. So now you can really have fun because you now know you are acting and you no longer take anything too seriously. You no longer go into the pit of pain and despair because the game is up. Illness is the expression of blocked energy and you know that you can now let it go.

So I do a mandala, almost with no purpose, no pressure, to rebalance from the release of the old energy. In other words no pressure to heal. Thus the mandala colouring is an opportunity to play with light in an open universe of experiencing. It simply becomes a matter of coming back to trusting your own Being. You can rebalance yourself at any time, and you do not actually have to do a thing, it does it on its own. Your body, your body of consciousness is waiting to do it. There is really nothing wrong with you unless you just happen to like playing that game. Your body consciousness is simply in the process of releasing blocked energy, and freeing and increasing the flow of life force as it is regenerating and evolving. You can build a health dynamic that will facilitate and make easier this transformation but the process and the timing is already taken care of.

You have been racing around, working, thinking, acting, restructuring. Your body has already healed itself but in a new place. Not in the old reality but in an entirely new place. Let it rebalance, and stop telling yourself that it is your 'fault' and you do not have the power and you cannot trust your body or think of it as powerful enough to heal itself without outside knowledge and skill. Heal yourself of the beliefs that you are unworthy and barely evolved from a "helpless beast nature". It is now time through your mandala sessions to just allow the changes to happen.

Your body is coming back to the natural state of being and the resulting changes that will occur from your colouring will give you enough trust in yourself to know that you can rebalance yourself. Your body consciousness is waiting to do what it knows it can. If you get involved in thinking about it, if any doubt creeps in, just take a deep breath and let it go.

Any time you want to rebalance yourself it is so easy. You don't have to know complex systems and techniques. A simplicity of spirit, the simplicity of Self is enough. It is fun. You don't have to think about it, just a few minutes, and let it happen. No more struggle. This is what use to be called "healing".

It is my view and experience that any system that does not keep it simple actually pushes wellness away somewhere else. People devise some complex system, put you through the maze, take your money, and you walk out thinking that you are not "good enough" to heal, not powerful enough, your beliefs and conviction are somehow flawed.

If you want to rebalance your body and mind, you do it simply. The less you try, the more effective it is.

You are a Divine Being and the Universe, through the infusion of the new energies and instantaneous availablity through the quantum field, have already put all the potential and the holographic blueprint of your perfected body form in place, and now it is a matter of being aware of this and allowing it to become your reality. So your only obstacle to wellness is the lack of your allowing yourself to heal.

The Art of Playing

A state of play in colouring your mandala is critical. It is a good idea to remember yourself as a child colouring in or even better try sharing a session of colouring with your children or grand children. See how they just enjoy doing it for its own sake and there is not expectation or big deal over any outcome whatsoever. They easily enter into a state of doing, and just as easily leave the activity and go onto something else. They look at what they have created when it is complete and mostly they are very pleased with it. There is a satisfaction and you may even hear a beautiful sigh of completion. Once you step into the state the colouring, play acts as the vehicle to take you into that state of being totally present .

The real key is to get into that state where you know nothing, so you can access everything, be open to anything, because it is all available. It is available not as a lesson with a purpose but as an experience to be enjoyed as it is.

So the optimum session is being lost in play again. A light heartedness that springs from just losing yourself (your self-conscious self).

Trusting Your Own Process

The New energy is like a great golden river of light and it flows by itself.   You cannot control it, you cannot speed it up or slow it down. It flows inexolorably and you are simply sinking into your heart space and trusting your inner process to guide you.

Trusting without prempting any particular outcome; watching, listening, trusting and surrendering. Surrender is relinquishing the refusal to let 'right' action move through you. In healing it means to quit focussing on the cure, quit fighting the disease, and awaken to your wellness. In life it means to quit looking for the bad or evil and awaken to good and beauty. It means to take full charge of your moods and to begin to live in flow by continually turning yourself towards feeling 'better', feeling grateful, feeling joy.

Do you realise that if you looked infinitely through telescopes or microscopes, you'd never see evil? Where do you see evil? When you look at each other. So we say let go. Surrender and begin looking for the Divine, the bigger of the more immediate picture, the larger or "now" view. How do you find it? You look with the expectation of beauty in front of you. You look at a tree, you look in the eyes and heart of a friend. You look to a sunrise or sunset, a tiny plant breaking through the earth, or to the stars. Why? Because the universe is perfection. You cannot add to perfection of the universe because it already is. What you can do is unencumber yourself from that which you have defined as imperfect. Whatever it is that you are afraid to lose is the very thing that is choking the life out of you. What are your guides telling you? Let go.

Free your heart and spirit and let the teaching begin. For the teaching and knowledge that will come will be remembrances. As you let go you return to your own personal light. What everything you are encountering is telling you is not only how to return to the light, but also how to be your own personal light, how to Shine.

It will be trust in yourself, and your willingness to stay open that will lead you to all your healing, no matter what the symptoms are.

Moving to the Heart

It is your mood that determines your bodily feeling of wellbeing and it is in wellbeing that you are aligned with health. Everything is energy and exists as vibration. Change the vibratory frequency you consciously project and you change, not only what you resonate with, but also the very state of matter or any energetic expression. Mandala colouring leads you easily into a state of consciousness whereby you become absorbed into the moments, into the momentum of stillness, a state of watching and being. You literally step out of your mind and into the activity, the circle, a new universe of nameless shape and developing colour and light. You step into yourself and out of the limitations your mind has habitually placed in front of you. And it is here that healing can occur because there is now allowance for the body to do its work, for the cells to do what they instinctively know they can do and that is to repair, to regenerate, and to clear that which is foreign unto itself. The mood you have generated will determine whether the cells move to wellness or further into disease.

The DNA strands can be seen of as brilliant sparks of light around you and they vibrate according what you consciously hold in your heart. Your state of "embracing readiness" as it were. DNA is in fact everywhere. It is the field of you that organizes itself into readable patterns of information (energy). It is a true reflection of your higher consciousness that is the director and decider of what is manifest in your field as form, and it is your wakefulness in this reality that determines what will be actively encouraged or discouraged in your physical body.

Science has shown us that the amount of winding or unwinding of the DNA is directly influenced by our intentional feeling, and especially through heart felt feelings of love, compassion, gratitude, peace and acceptance. These feeling tones known as 'Heartmind", in fact are the only states of mind that can at present be reliably demonstrated to produce observed changes in DNA. DNA is directly effected by your state of feeling-mind (consciousness).

These states collectively produce what is referred to a state of "coherence" since the electromagnetic waves generated by such states are characterised by frequencies with aligned peaks and oscillation. They are very powerful and their energy can be detected as extending out many feet from the body source.

The DNA particles vibrate in synchronicity with what your heart holds. These little sparks of light are always changing into the color of the core of their centre, circle or sphere of brilliant light. And when another color forms a new circle they change again. Every breath and every heartbeat is choice, and how you consciously connect to your heart is reflected in the colour, vibrancy, amplitude, and openness of these light string sequences. The more you maintain your core heart feeling as waves of love and compassion, the quicker these light particles will be able to change to provide the information you really want from them, ie. instructions to the cells for their perfected state. They actually unwind the DNA strings to release light. You are creating as you go, creating with every heartbeat, your creations, how your cells will develop, balance and organize, and your body's capacity to heal, will grow automatically. You do not need to know the full picture. Simply following your heart, and your inner sense of direction, is enough. Do what makes your heart sing, in every moment, again and again.

The light codes of DNA are simply the sparks of magnetism that so many of us are seeing around us. Magnetism equals Love. Magnetism just is, so in realizing that your 12 strands are magnetism, are love, and just is, you can also realize that this is where your experience of Oneness comes from. The centre of your heart, the eye of the spiral of your Being in your body, is in your heart.

Energy is always moving it is never still. Often you can feel stuck but in essence you never are. It is only the mind repeating the same scenario over and over. It is the illusionary reality that is stuck not the you in the Presence of I AM. By changing the thoughts or by moving from the mind into the heart, you move this forward. It is by no accident that the human heart when it feels pain wants to shut down. It is the teaching from birth for everyone that we protect ourselves from the world and it is the exact opposite from what should be done. Cruelty, hurtfulness. sadness, and depression, and in fact all negative action and expression are a result of having closed down the heart for self protection, and with it comes either loss of feeling or an over sensitivity and vulnerability in emotions.

Love changes how you can feel about anything. Love moves you to truth. The mind is always searching and searching for the answers but does not have the answers for healing. The heart does. The heart connects you to others and is the path to Source. Your heart knows the truth for that is how it was seeded. Seeds of fear cannot grow in the love that resides deep within the human heart for that love is always present even when you feel that it is not. If only you can step out of your mind, just for a moment and into the true place of love which is your heart. When you do you begin to get the vision of what you really need and the directions that will lead to more benevolent outcomes for yourself and those about you.

Your absorbtion in mandala colouring will take you to your heart centre , into the eye of the spiral , the I AM that you are, the mandala centre. The colours and their pattern will form a radiance of expression and will enliven your luminous field, your Shining. The mandala provides an implicit call from your heart for awakening that you have consciously initiated.

Summary: How it Works

When you open to the pure enjoyment of the process of colouring, choosing a design you resonate with, and the colours that draw themselves to you, you are activating a vibrational wave of information from your luminous field.

Your body wisdom impresses a design that is the highest common factor between its state at that time and the DNA informational patterns available to it in an infinite field of light/information potential present in your luminous matrix. It attracts a "best-match" vibrational sequence which is then called forth from the morphogenetic field.

On completion of the mandala, with sight, you would see that it immediately starts to spin and the resultant wave attracts a corresponding response from your expanded perfected blueprint, such that the body then begins to recalibrate the cell memories through the infusion of the incoming resonant wave of the new imprint. The mandala generates a specific wave signature and the only way the physical body can change is by altering its wave signature because the body (and all material substance) is composed of minute particles .

The key determinants of the speed and strength of the new download is the conscious clarity and focus of your awareness in Heartmind. That is, the extent to which you are able to let go of outcome and purpose, to surrender to alignment of feeling, trust in the whole process, and enjoy the experience.

Heartmind can only be experienced through love, compassion, joy, forgiveness, gratitude, peace, and harmony. This is why the efficacy of mandala drawing is primarily reflected in a childlike awareness of play and enjoyment for its own sake and with no other fix purpose except the experience itself. Remember, it is not about combating disease or infirmity, but about promoting your own wellness, energy, vitality, balance and all the feelings and sense that you experience as Heartmind. The clarity and strength of Heartmind is thus the prime determinant of the new DNA code activation. Your heart song literally is the signature that unlocks the information codes for your unique transformation. And it is through the Heartmind initiation that the most appropriate and relevant call to the information potential of your luminous field will be forthcoming.

The other most essential part of the transformation equation is your sense and your trust of your body processes. We hold so many beliefs that reflect the view of our body as an object rather than a sentient being. As you begin to work with the mandalas you are not only calling in new information. Your body will respond to these activations by requiring a new sense of "body presence", a new sense of its changing needs, and most importantly an increasing sense of its own consciousness as a unified grand community of living beings. A growing sense of the profound beauty and intelligence of ones body becomes an essential part of the transformation experience. You are a sovereign being whose consciousness has resided over the body and in not trusting your "subjects" you have unwittingly disempowered and subjected your community to decay and eventual demise. Giving back their freedom and trusting them to self govern, a wise leader will listen and provide whatever is needed to promote the wellbeing and the will of the people.

In the mandala colouring process you are essentially putting the mental mind aside to trust in the body and sense perceptions, and aligning with your Heartmind as it transmits an open wave to the DNA in the luminous field. Body being the source of 3D experience (not the mental logical mind), and heart being the eye of the circle and directly in contact with other dimensions of self (spirit) and the unlimited potential of Source.

CHAPTER 6   WALKING MY TALK: HEALING AND BELIEVING

I think it now becomes obvious how and why the drawing and colouring of a mandala might work in your transformation, your journey to wellness. Through breaking the inertia of a stalled and blocked belief systems, emotions and mind circuitry, the fundamental unimpeded allowance of energy movement of light codes initiates change in our energy system. A wave of illuminatory energy charge is radiated throughout our energy system triggering the necessary transformation for our balance in expanding consciousness.

If you think you can overcome, or better still, transcend the reality in which disease occurs, you can. If you think you can attain balance and vitality in your body you can. If you think you can remove genetic predispositions you can. You can do anything you can imagine. You just have to believe with all the imagination, feeling and knowing that you possess. You came here by choice to create the reality you prefer. It was your great and limitless love that brought together all the light particles that constitute who you are. It is your love, reflected through your Heartmind that can be directed towards anything you desire to become manifest in your existence. The community of love cells that make up your body only await your permission to do what they know how to do. And from the very Presence of the great love that you are, all that is ever needed already exists in your luminous field.

So as you create your mandalas you fashion a light song of coherent energy waves which resonates between your field and your form. This light filled song echoes a new wholesome manifestion of human form. And the dance begins in earnest, the dance of the transformation into a fully realised light consciousness brought about by your love filled knowing, and your belief in your own power to create. The mandala is an embodiment of you in the creating process.

With regards to my own health I had been asking my body to become completely healthy by recalling what its DNA blueprint holds as its most spectacular potential. I've asked it to bring forth everything that is Divine and allow it to be demonstrated both physically and non physically. My subconscious, non thinking, 'instinctual' mind, is more than capable of unraveling the code. I do not need to know any of it and in fact filling my mind with systems of objectification about how to become healthy will simply interfere with my free experience of what is happening.

One of the most important lessons for me has been not to focus on what I think I need to do and allowing things to transform. To see and flow with what is. Changes take time, they are a process that requires a foundation. It's easy to identify the quick fix or what we think is the "way", or to listen to what others say, yet my deeper self (guides, angels, guardians, the subconscious or whatever you wish to call it) moved me to where I needed to be and put me in the position to do what I need to do. After the fact it has been easy to see the foundation I have built and why it was required. None of what I have learned or gained has come from just one thing I had done, obtained or been. It has all come down to belief. How strong is my belief in the capacity of my body to heal and transform, how willing am I to listen to its prompting and trust its directions, and how willing am I to let go of all the other belief constructions that I have contrived, through my mind, that block the free flow of energy?

Walking My Talk

My motivation to write this book was so strongly guided by my familiarity and confidence in the power of mandalas to heal that I was ready and had all the chapters clearly in my mind within a few weeks and almost two years ago. I had written an outline and was ready to roll. This was going to be an enjoyable, smooth and easy creation, it was so clear in my mind. However, as it happened, for the next couple of weeks I started to feel a physical weakness begin to creep into my body. I felt dizzy and disoriented and I put it down to 'energy symptoms' which I had previously experienced on a number of occasions but which had dissipated after a couple of days. The symptoms got steadily worse until it reached the stage of chronic fatigue where I was finding it extremely difficult to get up off the bed. I had to focus on what I was doing and totally concentrate my will to move my body. I felt extremely fatigued, and my muscles seemed to be getting progressively weaker. With an increased sensitivity to light, if I walked outside in the garden I would have to close my eyes frequently in order to make progress. My ability to concentrate was poor and I had a 'spaced out' foggyness in the head. Rest and sleep did not seem to help. From my understanding of my symptoms I was experiencing full blown 'chronic fatigue'. It was not the usual passing symptoms that would be going away anytime soon. I knew that for some sufferers it had continued for years with little or no relief available with conventional medicine. My own view was that it is an energy disorder link to early emotional trauma. Regardless of the cause, the episode was so debilitating for me that it was time to do something about it.

You would have thought that using the mandalas would have occurred to me immediately but it took almost a month of experiencing this progressively debilitating physical state before the penny dropped. Going to a doctor was not an option for me. I searched my experience and knowledge, and the internet, for foods, herbs, and supplements, with no satisfactory outcome. I made strong affirmations, and looked into alternatives but none inspired my confidence. Eventually I heard an inner voice say loudly and clearly "Fool, what about mandalas?"

Feeling so weak and in a brain fog I chose my first mandala from a large selection (it turned out to be an open empty circle that impressed me) and I began to draw shapes and colour it in. It took a while with frequent rests but, much to my surprise, immediately after I had completed the session I felt a little better, a little energy had returned to my body. Day by day, each time I completed a mandala, I got progressively stronger and my immersion and enjoyment in the activity became easier as my symptoms eased. It took about two months for all the symptoms to leave me and by that time I had completed around 20 mandalas.

Well now I was ready to write the book, not only did I believe the mandalas worked, I now knew they did. I had experienced their magic first hand and irrefutably for me. But no, wait, my journey was not over, it had just begun. I started to get sick again. Not normally prone to flu or colds, I got the sneezes, headache, sweats, sore throat, the works. On such occasions I normally take no medication whatsoever and after three to seven days of symptoms my body has completed its work, with the help of rest, appropriate diet and liquid intake. However, this time, the symptoms did not go away and I got steadily worse. I developed bronchitis, sinus pain and blockage, allergic sneezing, asmatic breathing difficulties, and laryngitus. I was experiencing complete immunity breakdown. It got to the stage that every breath was an effort and there were times when I thought I was actually going to die. I had hardly the strength or capacity left to draw in the next breath.

Resolutely, I refused to seek medical help and I turned to my mandalas. Again, though at first in a very weak physical condition, and looking through eyes streaming with water, I pulled myself into a mandala session. The first mandala took a couple of sessions to complete but there was some enjoyment through the haze. Day by day, session by session, my health improved and another 20 odd mandalas and 3 months later I was totally clear. No medicine no healers, or outside intervention, just mandalas, and my normal responding to my body preferences and guidance for herbs and food. By now I was not quite as eager to dive straight in and write the book. Anything is possible and it turned out that it was.

It has been my view that the development of cancer in the body is strongly related to fear and fear maintenance. Thus although cancerous cells are continually present, our body can handle their removal and neutralise them, as long as we can maintain a predominately empowered state of being. Thus cancer becomes active when the emotional 'holding back' reaches a critical point for the individual. I believed that I was immune to cancer taking up residence in my body and it did not figure in my awareness as something I could experience. I had little fear of it but can see quite clearly how fear of it permeates our whole modern culture, and is especially perpetuated through attitudes associated with its diagnosis and the horrific stories both of treatment, painful suffering, and fatality, that are rampant today. The more its appearance has been feared the more prevalent it has become.

Almost a month after my immune system was back in balance I detected a growth in my left side a couple of inches from the navel. At first I thought it was just a tender spot that was hardened through muscular tension but over the next couple of weeks it had grown quickly to the size of a golf ball, along with increasing pain. I knew it was a tumor and I was starting to feel weaker and nauseas. Once again I took my treatment through mandala colouring. I chose again not to consult a doctor. I did not want to go through the tests and poking and prodding just to be told what I knew. I chose not to go through a 'health' system where I see people become sicker as soon as they receive their diagnosis. A system which gives little or no credence to the body's capacity to move to wellness. A system where the knife and poisoning (chemotherapy, radiation, and lethal drugs) of the body is seen as the only way to avoid suffering and death. A system that treats symptoms and gives little help or credence to the power of the patient nor the energetic basis of wellness and is biased towards reinforcing and duplicating other peoples' fears. Why would I want to do any of this? No, I know that my body has the natural capacity to deal with anything 'foreign' if I give it the chance. And so armed with the confidence of my recent experience with mandalas I knew they would provide the needed impetus for my wellness.

Thus, once again I embarked on a series of sessions along with eating healthily and some of the foods I knew to be associated with reduction of cancer. Twenty odd mandalas later, a couple of months, and the tumor and all the pain were gone. Unlike a medical diagnosis I can declare myself, not in remission, but as cancer free. My body has done with its presence and now has the instructions and experience to effect remedial action.

I speak of having cancer almost casually, but I did not have fear of it when the tumor appeared and my belief in the efficacy of mandalas and the power of my body to move to wellness was now unshakable. 'Cancer' was not cancer, but a growth that was expressing itself in my body, and when done, given the encouragement from me and access to its own data set from my luminous field, wellness and vitality are its natural state.

Therefore, after nearly 9 months and having completed 64 mandalas (See Figure 5), my journey of transformation was complete at this stage. Not only had I thrived after three major illnesses but also I had demonstrated to myself, in an irrefutable manner, how through the power of my belief in myself, in my body, and in the beingness of my luminous field, together with a so simple colouring session, I could restore the balance of my body.

Wellness is so much about Belief

My healing journey was about the beliefs I held and quantum healing is about learning to co-create with the Universe by being open to and listening to subtle energetic clues within my body-mind-spirit.

The word 'quantum' is used because of the degree of change and the instantaneousness of it. It describes the limitless availability of choice we have available to us when we open our minds to the fluidity of the Universe, rather than thinking of it and our bodies as solid unchangeable particles. It is truly about entering the mystery and trusting in the benevolent forces within us.

Although the concept is simple, navigating our old belief structure takes time and we often need to educate ourselves in order that we can become our own best healers. The clearing of physical symptoms comes from expanding our consciousness, releasing self-judgment, and shifting our perspective, to allow our body to navigate through the rebalancing that can naturally, instinctively take place. It is essentially being able to totally accept the unshakable belief that we hold the power to move to wellness.

The Dismantling of Belief

I am saying that all physical disease, affliction, pain, discomfort, imbalance is a reflection of beliefs we hold that are perpetuating untruths about ourselves. We are holding and maintaining beliefs about ourselves that are disempowering, that deny in some way the truth of our origin, belonging, worthiness, and power to create. We hold within explanations of unconscious, old unresolved energies of emotionally charged memories that are solidified by beliefs about ourselves and that negate, in one way or another,

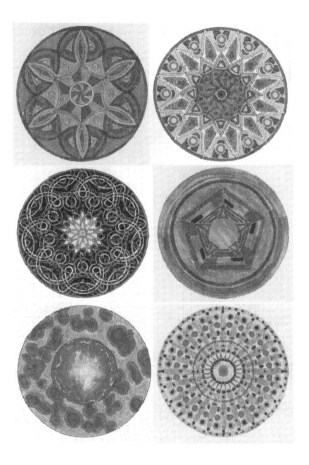

Figure 5

Examples of my own completed Mandalas. Second down on the right is a crop circle and third on the left is based on a simple circle design and was completed during the cancer phase of my healing journey.

the fact that we are love incarnate, that we are One in and One with the Source of All That Is.

Instead we could be telling ourselves that we really do know who we are, and that we are creators of all that we have, can and do experience. That all the information and resource for our total wellness is available, at this moment, through our luminous field. If we can understand that we experience an energy flow from our field through the navel vortex ('gut reaction') and which flows up and sits under the heart. Pressure from the block of this flow impinges on heart from triggered memories in brain (left side), and if too painful to be taken up into the heart, forming a loop and is expressed through dreams, fantacies, and unconscious, instinctual reponses (defense mechanisms). Finally the unresolved energy builds and is reflected in the body by painful and debilitating symptoms. The body is like a last resort to get our attention.

We permanently free the energy by the acknowledgement and release of the beliefs that prevents the energy from flowing freely through the heart. And we have seen that resolution and disappearance of symptoms comes from simple recognition, viewing from heartmind, which releases the emotional charge. The symptoms have to be felt in order to unblock the energy that is locked in fear, anger, etc.

So the only real work we need to consciously engage in is a step by step process of dismantling and discarding all the beliefs we hold that disempower us and speak to us untruths about the nature of who and what we are. This in itself does not need to be arduous. Just a simple recognition of any untruth about ourselves and a taking back in, with feeling and compassion, will release the blockage by our acceptance of a fuller appreciation of ourselves and who we are. We do not even have to look for the blockages. The beliefs are reflected in all the doubts we have about our own power and the power of our body to restore the necessary balance and the extent to which we can respond to our body's prompting for what it needs to support the changes it is making. Recognise and attend to the removal of the doubts and the energy blocks are released

The crux centres around the dropping of inappropriate belief and adopting belief that maintains a reality of health, wellness, and wholeness. Jesus always asked of those he was about to heal "Do you believe". He was so convinced of his own and everyones power to be well if they wanted to, and so in the power of the absolute truth of his knowing he was able to hold the space for anyone to step into wellbeing. But once they were not in his presence he knew that, in order to maintain their wellness, they would have to believe in their own power, and their unwavering connection to the Divine all knowing, all compassionate, all creative Presence. It was, in those days, referred to as "faith in God". The power of the placebo (sugar pill) centres around the power of belief that the treatment or the medicine being given really works. So a no treatment condition, more often than not, has more success than all kinds of other treatment, if the patient is strongly convinced that it will.

Overcoming Doubt

From time to time throughout my healing journey I had to confront and let go of doubts about my power and the truth of my inner prompting. The pressure of doubt and need to seek conformation became particularly relevant when the growth appeared and I knew that a tumor was growing inside me.

Perhaps I really needed to see my doctor and get tests and some confirmation. I had to remind myself, however, that generally an illness will really begin to gather momentum right at time of diagnosis. If doctors can catch things in the early stages they will often talk you into full blown illness. Medical professionals can take simple symptoms of energy blockage and scare the patient to death over illnesses that are in other peoples bodies. Patients are convinced to push against their body which wants to move towards natural wellbeing. Illnesses in our society are increasing as we become increasingly engaged with disease and ill health rather than wellbeing. We are often embarassed into tests and treatment and I have never heard a physician say that my body has the resources to right itself.

Health is all about energy flow and who is it that knows how it is flowing in your body? I know, I can tell in the early subtle stages whether I am flowing towards wellness, or pushing against it. I don't need your tests or your cure. Our medicine is always looking for the cure when it does not even know the cause. The cause is energy and the shift of energy is accomplished through thought and emotion (feeling).

What mandalas do is put you into a state of feeling better which is in energy alignment with wellness. The colouring experience facilitates your shift to wellness consciousness and the resultant colour vortex symphony does the rest.

All negative sensations are about how energy is flowing in your system. All illnesses start with a sensation of negative emotion. First it is a sensation of, then it is the manifestation of energy that does not feel good. At any point, whether it is a mild negative sensation, or an early showing on tests or whether it is a fully progressive illness, it does not matter because I have found that at any point, if I can stop and relax in it, instead of pushing against it, this is where colouring a mandala really helps and my body will right itself. It allowed me to make a shift in consciousness and for my body to make the changes it needed to make.

It is not about illness jumping into my body but about me holding wellness out. I don't get ill because I focus on cancer or immune deficiency, or chronic fatigue every day, I get these and other indications of energy blockage because I find things to worry about, to push against, because I feel guilty, blameful, or angry, I disrupt the flow of experience through my heart centre. If I listen to others who reinforce the idea of fear and powerlessness, that I am wrong or do not have the right knowledge or tools or skill, in that moment that I am convinced by them that somehow I am inadequate, I have allowed them to point me in the direction of illness.

How was the mandala colouring so successful in releasing my symptoms? Purely and simply it was successful because I knew it was going to be. I took my knowing of the intelligence of my body, my community of cells. I accepted that I came here as a Divine being and that it was my love and my desire to be here that first magnetised all the adamantine particles of pure light to form a vehicle that I could live in. That the cells thus congregated, connected and integrated to form in a vessel for the light of my consciousness to experience the third dimension in the most benevolent and fulfilling manner it could, based on the evolutionary potential of physical matter and the dictates of the journey I had planned for it. Each cell has its memory, not just of a history of genetic experience, but also of a potential to expand its experience and thereby make an evolutionary shift in its vibratory rate.

I came to alter the nature of matter through my cellular transformation based on a new blueprint for humankind. All I needed to do was to provide the environment for the cells to do their work of transformation by removing all the energy blockages to their evolutionary shift. And the only stumbling blocks to that evolution is the beliefs I or my ancestors have held that negate the knowing that I am One in and One with the Source of All that Is.

So essentially all I had to do was to get out of my own way. To no longer accept any idea or belief that I needed anything else but my loving appreciation of my cell community in order for transformation (healing) to take place. To understand that the bodily affliction was the playing out of energy blockages in dense matter and that it was the cells capacity to handle these that needed to be recognised and allowed to run its course without interference from me. Without me trying to control proceedings and project the unkind lies onto them that they needed help because they could not do what they were designed to do.

My work was to provide the best environment in order for them to do their job and so the key was first to believe in them and secondly to provide the love, gratitude and joyful experience of being alive. Of course providing physically, through diet, water, exercise, rest and comfort was also part of it since it reflects my care for my body and my pleasure in the experiences it provides me with. But the big requirement was to do so with ease and trust and not do it with a load more fears of trying to do the right thing. Simple, slow, gentle and kind. For example, enjoying what I eat with no stops or inhibitions. Eating what I got an immediate "yes" to and not getting drawn into the old patterns and hassles of whether it is "good" for me.

Summary

Healing comes from being in a greater state of allowing or a greater willingness to be receptive. Colouring mandalas causes you to soften your resistence to allow the wellbeing that would have been there otherwise anyway. "Cure" or remedy to any affliction is always and only about allowing wellbeing. All the organs and the cells of the body know what to do to maintain the balance. If they are not being denied access or being hindered by the accumulation of the disbeliefs in our own power, which disrupts the flow between the cells and the universal flow, health and wellbeing are assured. The mind is seeded with fear and confusion and will always attempt to replay a scenario over and over trying to find another ending. Howvever, this is illusion for the ending can never be any different from what actually did happen unless you choose a reality that is different.

Be clear that I am not advocating here that you should ignore other healing regimes or drop whatever you are doing for health and replace it merely with mandala practice. Each of us has a healing journey and health is as much a developing relationship with your body consciousness as it about any particular practice. The normal medical route may be a necessary part of an individual's journey. A dietry alternative can also be quite effective. What is critical is your empowerment in the entire journey. I am advocating, however, that listening and responding to your own promptings is crucial for wellness.

I have used mandalas almost exclusively for my healing transformation journey because I knew that they would be successful, and did this with the conviction based on the strength of my experience. How much the experience becomes part of your process is of course up to your own discovery.

For the journey to wellness it does not seem to matter what type of medicine is administered, the common denominator that seems to matter is that the one receiving it believes that it is the best. Whatever it takes to assist you to allow what you really want to happen. Instead of shutting down the heart from the pain, the heart chakra should be opened so that love pours through you in order to heal what you have taken on and now decided to release. You are on a healing journey as much as you are on a life journey. You cannot heal what you will not look at. Your mind will imprison you in pain while your heart knows the way to heal that pain.

It is our mind that through beliefs tries to find answers for energy blockages. Once an explanation is found that feeds and satisfies the mind it rests, and in that rest is the illusion that balance has been restored. However, energy blocks are emotional in nature and are the domain of the heart. The heart knows about emotion and it is the heart that releases and transforms the energetic expression and the blocked energy flow. It is the heartmind that knows how to heal emotion and thus the appropriate energy flow for the health of the body.

CHAPTER 7 BLUEPRINT FOR CHANGE: MANDALA ACTIVATION PROGRAMME

We have said that absolutely everything you need for your complete experience of wellness is within you. Not only does all the potential, the energy, and the information, required for everything you could possibly dream of, is present now in your luminous field, your body knows exactly where to go to get the information for its transformation. Thus our change is about trust in all that we are. No longer trying to work everything out, attempting to contrive plans for survival and to protect ourselves from harm by continually trying to project into the future what might happen and how to guard against it. Transformation is about becoming fearless. Not even fearing death because you know that it is an illusion and that, because you are connected to Source and All That Is, there will be no more loss than stepping out of used clothes. When you can truly and totally trust your body, and Earth, and the Universe, you will be totally healed and living in the wellness stream.

It does not mean that you will not have body symptoms, for these are indicators of change, but they do not have to be drastic, or acutely painful, or debilitating. They will serve you because you will no longer be afraid of them nor treat them as indicating something is 'wrong', as invaders, as alien to you.

It is all about change and we are beings on the move, in the process of an evolutionary shift, and when you enter the experience of the mandala you are inviting accelerated change in all levels of your experiencing self. From your very first colouring session you are stepping out of the 3rd into the 5th dimension, out of linear time into the Now. The mandala becomes a spiral vortex which, quite easily, naturally, and literally draws you simultaneously into yourself and 'out' into your sense of Oneness.

The transformation to the 5th dimension is the tranformation to the NOW. Though in the 3rd dimension we experience everything as relative and as contrasting, in others words as a duality, there is no such experience in the 5th, 'stepping into' your mandala creating is stepping into the simultaneous ebb and flow of change and expansion, where coming together is created and separation dissolves. Peace, love, joy, abundance, and freedom lives in that time and space that you are tapping into within yourself. In fact in this 5th dimensional experience, time and space become fluid and illusionary. In the now moment, through the easy letting go of attachments and identities, as you become immersed in the experience, Presence begins to pervade your experience in your session, the feeling of "Yes" to everything, a subtle but indefinable 'pleasantness' and calm, a quiet expectation of goodness and benevolence. Mandalas put you onto a natural flow of Now. You lose your resistance to what is 'out there'. You sit in peace with yourself.

So by entering the the spiral you move out of the mind and into your heart, and move into expanded consciousness whereby other potential for change, for transformation becomes possible.

Stepping into Change.

We human beings, by our very nature, are curious, sense and sensation seeking creatures. We thrive on novelty and wither, atrify and shrivel up with boredom, apathy, and sameness. We find great joy in pleasant surprises and we switch off from the repetitive, the 'humdrum'. It is threat and fear that teaches our children to withdraw from life and it is our insecurities which push us to accept only what we know, and fear what we do not. We learn to seek and prefer a sense of certainty rather than a sense of adventure. Our need for certainty flies in the face of everything we are. Everything in the universe is in continual movement. Sometimes your reality can feel fairly organised and simple but more often than not, in these times, everything about and around you can seem totally complex, out of order, falling apart, in total and continual flux and chaos both within and without. This is especially true when you try to put any sense to it with your thinking. In fact in these times it is impossible to make any sense of it whatsoever. This chaotic state is in fact a very good sign to us that what we have asked and yearn for is in the process of becoming. Change is here now and it is only our fear of not knowing and not feeling in control, and the resistance habits for change we have maintained, that make it so uncomfortable. Change is inevitable and it is why we came here and what we have called for. The problem is simply, how can we enhance and expand our comfort in the process of change?

Our energy has got stuck, and blocked the flow of life force. We have resisted change, have been afraid of it, afraid of the unknown. You may have felt many times that you needed to make a change in your life but somehow always come up against a wall. Often you make attempts to change but in one way or another you have met discouragement, and fall back into lithargy, blaming either yourself for some lack, or others for lack of support. The good news is that there is a way out and it is very simple.

The Chinese have a saying "The best way to avoid evil is to make energetic progress in the good". What is meant is that if you want to change from a "bad" habit, in this case lack of movement in the direction you would prefer to go, that is, towards wellbeing, then you need to put some energy into the direction you want to go. So in our case I am saying it will benefit you to allowing mandalas to befriend you and you to befriend them, because they will move you into the comfort of movement, expansion, and change.

Programming for Change

So how much is enough energy to making a real difference in where you are headed with your mandala experience into wellbeing?

Change is the journey and there is no end to expansion.

We came here into a time point of complete change, a vortex of an evolutionary leap. The old duality consciousness is dying human systems of government, finance, law, medical, technological, science and education, social and class, attitudes and values are all crumbling, all going, disintegrating into a melting pot of change. There is nowhere to go. The past is obsolete providing little to rely on and the future appears as a blank canvas. But it is in this apparent chaos that the new unpredictable is possible and will be born.

So it is about living in change, continuous unfolding and expansion of Self, living in the moment, and trusting what is birthing within and around you. Nothing set, the future is to be born out of the now and is to be totally an individual matter. Each of us is changing by a Law of our own transformation, our own ascension. There are waves of energy that we are living in but the particular expression of our unfolding is each our own, and springs from our full conscious participation in living all that we can be.

The Number of Mandalas for Symptom Removal

So to the question of how many mandala sessions are required to effect changes that bring our energetic bodies back into alignment ? How many mandalas and how often will be enough to complete the information download for the activation of the wellness blueprint. The simple answer is that it is an intuitive process and therefore the number of sessions and their timing is entirely an individual matter. When you are open to the potential of the changes then you set in motion a complete chain of events in the natural unfolding of you. Intuitively you will receive prompts to enter into a mandala session. You will "feel" like doing one. How quickly you respond within the constraints of your daily activities, is up to you but it is clearly efficacious to do it as soon as is practical for you.

Again you will know when you have completed your phase of "healing". Along with the disappearance of the symptoms there will be a sense of completion and a tangible feeling of increased ease in your body. There, of course, will be other times, other levels and other energetic movements you will be required to engage in but it will be clear to you when you are prompted to do further alignments. Sometimes you may not even feel any uncomfortable body sensations but be moved to make some alignment through colouring.

A Grande Design

Having said this, there is a pattern, and grande design, that is at work in the process of DNA download, especially where the physical body is concerned.

It is a beautiful, regulated design based in sacred geometric laws of physical manifestation. It is here in the specification of an implicit download pattern that I was first impressed to write this book.

Remember I have said that I kept getting a prompt to write this book based on the number "8" and the configuration of "8 x 8". The number 64 was clearly a part of this but the only thing at that time I could relate it to was the I Ching. This Chinese oracle is known as "The book of changes". I had studied and used the oracle frequently, many years previously, and perhaps it was no accident that it was Carl Jung, my mandala mentor, who had introduced it to me.

The I Ching is a very ancient system, that lays out a design of creation in which influences of nature have different properties that effect change (hexigrams), and these are constructed from base elements consisting of a combination of three (trigrams) "atoms". The system is comprised of 64 hexigrams, being all the possible combinations of the trigrams in pairs (see Figure 6).

The way in which the Book of Changes works is rather like a electrical circuit that reaches into all situations. The circuit only affords the potentiality of lighting but it does not give light. However, when contact with a definite situation is

The I Ching Blueprint

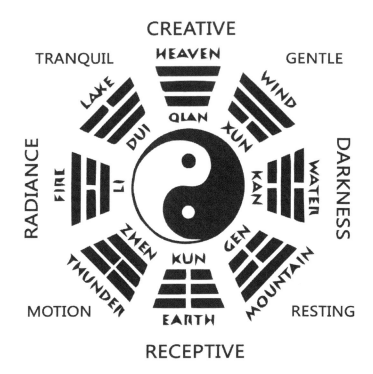

Figure 6

Figure 6 shows the basic I Ching coding system of natural cycles with the eight basic trigrams around the circle of creation. Top, bottom left, and right are at balance points in the energy waves of change cycle, whereas the four diagonal trigrams are at points of transition.

established through the seekers question, the 'current' is activated, and the given situation is illumined by which of the 64 hexigrams is divined. In other words when the seeker has made their selection the oracle 'plugs' them in. Analogously choosing your mandala plugs you in to a particular coded information light packet in your new DNA blueprint.

My own life purpose has been centered around personal change and self empowerment. In my early teens I studied writings about travelling the "spiritual path", the requirements and demands of the "initiate", and the nature of consciousness. For many years I have been enthusiastic about the possible link between the I Ching and DNA. While such a relationship is beyond the scope of this book, what this interest did do is point me in the direction of personal change and DNA and led me to the discovery that the DNA of our physical body has 64 codons.

In other words if we take the four basic elements of DNA, guanine, adenine, thymine, and cytosine, and arrange them in all the possible combinations of pairs, there are 64. It is interesting that only 22 have been active in the human body so there is already the possibility that there is much scope for a new evolved and "improved" physical form based on all 64 codons.

So here we have the number 64 (8x8) as central to the structure of physical DNA and the nature of change cycles reflected in the I Ching.. One of the properties of the number 64 is that we can take all the numbers inclusive of 1 to 64 and rearrange them to form a "magic square". That is a 8x8 matrix in which all the numbers horizontally, vertically, and diagonally add up to the same number (see Figure 7). This number just happens to be 260 which is the number of days of gestation for the human birth cycle. So 64 and 260 are vital bits of information about complete and completing cycles of human life.

During my own healing journey I had numbered my mandalas and recorded the date completed for each (for some of my completed mandalas refer to Figure 5). To my surprise and delight I coloured 64 mandalas after the ending of my third chronic disease cycle, for which there was a full sense of completion. Furthermore, the period from the first to the last mandala wasexactly 260 days. There was nothing randomly

Figure 7

8 x 8 Magic Square

								260
64	2	3	61	60	6	7	57	260
9	55	54	12	13	51	50	16	260
17	47	46	20	21	43	42	24	260
40	26	27	37	36	30	31	33	260
32	34	35	29	28	38	39	25	260
41	23	22	44	45	19	18	48	260
49	15	14	52	53	11	10	56	260
8	58	59	5	4	62	63	1	260
260	260	260	260	260	260	260	260	260

Figure 7 Shows the 'Magic Square' for the number "64" in which the sum of the numbers in all the rows, columns, and diagonals total 260

happening here. As I reached the end of this particular journey a larger design was clearly at work.

Subsequently, for others I have advised who have taken the mandala colouring as a dynamic in their life, a sense of completion is strongly present with or without immediate change in symptoms, when 64 drawings are completed. Though healing and changes, physically, emotionally, mentally and creatively, can occur with any number of mandalas completed, a quite marked stepping up of frequency and deepening of satisfaction is often felt having completed a 64 mandala cycle.

If your belief is strong and clear enough you can do anything. I had demonstrated to myself this and for good measure some months after my healing walk I was given a quick, concrete and irrefutable demonstration. I started to have very sharp pains in the upper abdomen, and a little nausea. Listening to my body my immediate impression was that of gall stones. I set to with a mandala and after five days and five mandalas later I quite literally experienced a pop in the region of my pain. Thirty minutes latter I had a quick and vigorous bowel movement that felt like expelling sand. I looked, and a grey course grit was clearly visible in the pan. Even though confident in efficacy of the mandalas I still feel the miracle of the rapidity of this demonstration as if a laser had blasted the gall stones, and the fact that I had seen the results with my own eyes.

Thus the mandalas have both gross and subtle effects both in short and longer term recovery.

Sixty four days appears to be enough for you to effect a significant shift in both your feeling and your conscious comprehension of what it is like to observe yourself, be a watcher, and be in tune enough to really listen to your body. It will be sufficient to establish the knowing and confidence in your power to begin to lead yourself to wellness, health and balance through definite, self initiated action, and your own creative capacity.

Summary

It is highly recommended that if you enjoy the activity that you include it as one of the tools in your self empowerment regime. Repeated exposure to the code and geometry of the new human blueprint initiates an activation integration dynamic. To accommodate the amplification of its data we must recalibrate to its frequency which initiates the 'cleansing'. As electromagnetic frequencies are downloaded into the endocrine system via circuitry the body emits alternate frequency resonant with the unique mandala configurations and an 'immortal' directive such that the old reality patterns will not be able to hold their molecular structure. Mandalas like the DNA are light receptive portals. Our body is filled with light receptive portals.

The DNA responds instantaneously to the "coherent' feelings and high frequency light initiated through the mandalas. It unravel, opens up when in the presence of love and closes in the presence of fear, and fear related emotions.

Our conscious process is to unravel the mind and let the feeling out. Feeling is locked in the binding thoughts. We step out of them by playing with them, playing with the words, the ideas, the thoughts, images and releasing them. They cannot trap you if you do not take them seriously any more. If you no longer try to be "right", nor try to control the apparent complexity of everything. Through mandala drawing, you move into the simplicity and joy of now. You will touch the gentle, open, connection to all that you are. You will be in the balance of feminine receptiveness and masculine power of expression. As the feelings are released from the thought in your play, there is an opening and expansion of a knowing resonance, harmony, and natural blending. Some call it Divine Beingness, you could point to it as Heartmind, but it needs no definition. You will know it as your own whatever is said about it. It is in essence the seed of a most beautiful, perpetual wave motion of lovingness to your self and your reality

CHAPTER 8   CREATION CODES AND APPLICATIONS

Mandalas are vortices through self to Self. They provide a template for consciousness movement through the physical, etheric, emotional, and mental levels of energy frequency of self to the higher frequencies of Self. They provide access to and lead the awareness into a more primal and formative level of Being beyond language and mental mind construction. They are Power templates mimicking the energetic characteristics of the singularity. The singularity with a toroidal, two fold action, of the Flow outlined in Chapter 1. Thus for all mandalas there is the pull (attraction) of perception and consciousness to the centre of the circle, the Source of Being, and a simultaneous expansion of flow out from the centre in all directions towards the "infinite boundary" of creation. The same dual forces that make up a galaxy, or the smallest particle.

Thus mandalas contain these forces implicit in them, and their action on our consciousness becomes undeniable once we intentionally engage with them. At the very least they draw you into a space of mental stillness and they open the portal to the subconscious and superconscious self, making available new knowledge, insights, and experiences as well as providing access to new blueprints and energy activation codes which have been, until this time, almost inaccessible.

The mandala works with the two movements from the outside towards the centre, and from the centre to the expanding infinity. From the conscious self to the Source (higher Self), and back from the Self to the self. Thus they provide for the possibility of wholeness that leads to Wellness, balance, and resting aliveness.

The glyph of the circle with the dot in the middle stands for the blueprint of Wholeness, and as the master pictogram for all mandalas.

Patterns of Creation

To simply look into one of these sacred circles that you have chosen and coloured is to enter into the heart of your being. It is to encounter aspects of yourself that are one with the sacredness in which the whole of reality is bathed.

No matter what may be going on in your life right now, simply looking at your mandala can bring you into that still place within you. In this stillness, you can discover how blissful it can be to live in the sacred wholeness of your deepest being.

You will also begin to experience that wise part of yourself that can provide you with the answers to every challenging issue you are facing - whether you are experiencing sadness, depression, anger, problems at work, or difficulties in your relationships with others.

As we have seen, in the effortless effort of a mandala session, healing happens. We move to a middle point of awareness, where mental mind cannot go, and the innocent, playful, delighting feelings emerge.

Sacred Geometry and the Mandala Experience

The mandala as circle pattern used for the process outlined in previous chapters is a powerful activator of creation and change.

Such patterns and configurations are formative in the very creation of our physical world and are what is referred to as sacred geometry, where crystaline and organic forms are seen to have clear geometric structures at the very basis of their blueprint.

Furthermore, their power and familiarity is never more clear or certain to us than when we gaze at the configurations of crop circles. These seem to have an allure and familiarity that defies description.

All life emerges from the same Source Intelligent, unconditionally loving, infinitely creative and represented in the universal language of sacred geometry. It is recognized on a cellular level by all beings. It is the language of consciousness, a language that speaks of the undeniable Oneness of all things. The whole Universe is a single wave pulse that expands and multiplies in all directions and dimensions creating an unlimited variety of vibrations. Sacred geometry corresponds to these vibrations. Interacting and meditating on sacred geometry symbols creates a higher vibration in our consciousness. Sacred geometry acts as a portal (a passage way to higher consciousness). Our mind opens to the vibrations of that particular symbol thus 'entraining' (synchronizing the wave forms) of our awareness to vibrate to that particular wavelength. The sacred form acts as a trigger to lead our higher mind, if the mental mind is not busy. It facilitates our transcendence into Oneself.

Sacred geometry is an ancient science, a sacred language, and a key to understanding the way the Universe is designed. It is the study of shape and form, wave and vibration, and moving beyond third dimensional reality. It is the language of creation, which exists as the foundation of all matter, and it is the vehicle for spirit. It has been called the "blueprint for all creation," the "harmonic configuration of the Soul," the "divine rhythm which results in manifest experience." Sacred geometry has the capability to balance human energy fields, open the pineal gland, and it contains a complex informational system that can be used to access healing and growth in many dimensions of experience. It 'speaks' a Language of Light

The Language of Light is already pre-coded into every cell of our body. We all have these light codes in us pre-coded to awakening. These dormant codes are awakened by light filled sacred geometric shapes, the Language of Light. Sacred geometry is a way of receiving information and energy to accelerate the shifting consciousness and the ascension process. As the Language of Light flows from "higher" dimensions into our world it holds an electromagnetic inscription encoded in certain geometric shapes, many of which occur in the mandalas used for our purposes. They are directly teaching your cellular level, and are 'heard' by your DNA.

Crop Circles

Crop circles are one of the most profound and mysterious phenomena of the modern age. They have had a powerful effect on thousands of people who have witnessed and studied them through the years.

Even to the most casual observer, the crop formations are eye-catching and beautiful. To mathematicians they represent the presence of an original and profoundly deep intelligence. To an ever-expanding community of spiritual seekers they symbolize that our planet is reaching a decisive stage of evolution. As well, they indicate contact with kindred earth energies, spirits, or devas, or kindred extraterrestrial beings whose communications are emerging at this time to assist us through this critical point in our planet's and our species' history.

These patterns have such a hypnotic effect on so many but what makes these crop circles (mandalas) so powerful? During reconstruction of the different crop circles you will see repeatedly perfect ratios, and formulas being printed on the earth. The shapes appear to work deep inside us in such a way that they enable us to do and feel things that we were unable to access before.

The Sacred Geometry within these formations is recognized by the subconscious, since all living creatures consist of geometrically shaped elements. The Golden Ratio is such an example and frequently appears in crop circles. The purpose of this 'supernatural' communication through mandalas appears to guide humankind in its evolution to a higher level of consciousness.

Essentially, crop circles are visible expressions of energy forms, and these forms are conscious and vibratory in nature. Unaltered photos of crop circles contained a code that systems in distress required to rejuvenate themselves. Simply put, each crop circle acts as a piece of 'software' that tells the 'hard drive' of a biological system how to rebuild itself. Photos or accurate drawings of these energy imprints, from their original designs in the fields have been used to send healing to any system in distress. A person, a tree, a forest, a river and the results can be incredibly positive.

If used responsibly, and always with the intent 'for the highest good of all', crop circles photos and drawings can be a trigger that activates these symbols. The crop designs have been used in homeopathy and other water coding procedures and now I include them in my collection of mandalas for a similar purpose, to trigger DNA codes for the reactivation of cellular memory.The crop circle drawings can be seen as carrying the missing code that the ecosystem, or person in treatment needs to revitalize the entire affected organism like a computer requiring a new chip in order to boot the rest of the system.

We now begin to understand why the crop patterns are coded with such geometric precision, and why they have such a mesmerizing effect on the human psyche. Because they contain natural frequencies and are designed upon the same crystalline patterns as our very own cells, they are mirrors of ourselves. They also begin to show us just why the ancients were so attached to practicing sacred geometry, why they encoded it into their building practices, and why Buddhist mandalas are said to impact the subconscious mind to such an effective degree. Crop circles are showing us a very old science, a natural science, and once again, it is accessible to all as shown throughout this book.

When you look at a crop circle, you are bringing healing to yourself. They have a powerful purpose and they can bring profound peace and healing. Throughout my own wellness journey I ensured that both open and concentric circles, sacred geometry, especially the 'flower of life' configurations, and crop circle designs were always made available in my resource of mandalas from which to make my choice for any given colouring session. I therefore strongly recommend the reader to consider them in their own mandala drawing resource.

Some Applications of Mandalas

Since completing my first journey with colouring mandalas I have conducted a number of group and individual sessions. The results and repercussions for participants have been many and varied. Some reporting, immediately following their session, heavy fatigue followed by a long, deep, relaxing sleep and waking totally refreshed. Others feeling head pressure and headache followed the next day by distinct feelings of freedom and joy, while others were fatigued for two or three days needing more rest than usual. Still others have found a problem that had been perplexing them was suddenly resolved either during or subsequent to their session. Most find the colouring enjoyable, absorbing, and even addictive.

Individuals who voluntarily decide to continue the practice have shared many different and varied experiences that they attribute to the mandalas.

Here are a few examples of how mandalas have been used.

1. One therapist uses the mandala colouring to centre herself and to tune in to the energies within herself and those she will be working with in self awareness workshops she conducts.

2. Another uses them before her life coaching session and whenever she needs to prepare for a client and is unsure how to procede.

3. Another uses them for an extension of her healing practice to tune into her own body sensing in order to be more sensitive and accurate with her clients.

4. Talya at age 9 years decided to colour a mandala for our cat Ra who was diagnosed with subcutaneous emphysema, which occurs when gas or air is present under the skin as a result of acute lung infection. The vet did not expect him to survive and so he was with us for possibly his final hours. She coloured two mandalas and placed each under the cat's front paw as he lay almost motionless. He did not move his paws and the next morning none of the "skin popping" remained. He had recover quickly and completely.

5. Georgia aged 10 years from time to time can be an emotional "drama queen" after a day at school, now she has a release. She takes herself off to her bedroom and colours in a mandala and comes out energised, centred, refreshed, and, as she says, feeling "herself".

6. Two young adults, breaking long term drug abuse are finding that regular mandala sessions are having a decided effect on centering and helping them to strengthen their resolve as well as open themselves up to new possibilities in their lives.

7. We have used mandalas to energise water. A mandala is chosen and coloured with the intentions of energy, love and purity. The mandala is then pasted to a large water container and filled with water for a couple of hours in sunlight or overnight. The water tastes sweet and contains the appropriate crystaline form generated from the frequency of the mandala.

8. We have used mandala colouring at gatherings with friends and family. Children love it and the settling effects on parents and adults, and the change in their demeanor and conversation, can be quite remarkable.

9. Many of my clients frequently use mandalas as a shared activity with their children. They report some significant harmonious changes in their relationships. Mandalas are powerful images to share with others. Through them we can share our inner realities with family and friends in honest and open ways, whenever we choose, and by this encourage our loved ones to share with us their depths   as   well.

    Just as a crop circle imprinted in a field in England can provide and energetic to the whole earth as well as to you and I in another timespace from its original creation, so too a mandala provides an energetic available to all. Healing self becomes healing All. Each one of us can add immediately to the transformation dynamic of all Humankind. And thus you really do become the change you have been searching for.

Sharing a Mandala Session

A word to "would be' mandala practicioners. Share in a mandala colouring time casually and playfully, but I would advise not to teach this as a modality of healing to others until you have completed a full 64 mandala sequence and have demonstrated their power for transformation in yourself first hand. We are living in the New energies and as such to be real and effective any technique is best shared from a point of view that knows. In other words the process should be active, alive and real both in your experience and in your knowing. This is a fundamental principle of the energies we are now living in. Being real, being authentic and being confident. If you try to fake or pretend to yourself that it works without experiencing its power then you are sharing nothing and it will not work for you. If you share with full integrity you offer the gift of your truth and your knowing, free of doubt and contrivance. This in itself makes available an enlivened accelerated opportunity for another to step into their own power of healing.

Consciousness Creates Our Body

If you expand your consciousness when you read a book you get more understanding, if look around you without trying to classify everything you get more awareness, and when you wake up consciously you have more wakefulness. And there is an ocean of pure vibrant consciousness inside each one of us. And it is right at the base of mind, right at the base of thought, and at the source of all matter.

All matter originates and exists only by virtue of a force which brings the particle of an atom to vibration and holds this most minute solar system of the atom together. Behind this force is the existence of a conscious and Intelligent Mind which forms the matrix of all matter.

The solidity of the world seems indisputable like a fixed thing you can see and touch. Your body is also reassuringly solid but modern physics has assured us that this solidity is a mirage. All of physical matter, everything we have around us is the result of a frequency and if you amplify the frequency the structure of the matter will change.

You are a self contained system, a hologram, and everything within is an expression of that hologram. Every part of that holographic picture is a smaller version of the whole (eg spiral galaxy). So reality is all connected and when you look at one small part you can see things about other parts. The entire whole is contained in the part so you cannot really divide reality up because you are cutting up a hologram. You cannot find where one particle is because it is always a reflection of all particles.

In a hologram the entire pattern is whole and complete unto itself. If you were to take any portion of this whole out and examine it closely you would see the entire pattern repeating itself (fractals) again and again. Anywhere in this pattern if we were to change one small aspect on any one of these infinite number of holograms, that change would be reflected throughout the entire system. A change in one cell effects a change in all cells.

The substance of the universe is consciousness thus it is behaviour that is important. Fear is a very slow, dense vibrational state and the more you buy into fear (and the whole of our current dying global society is structured to make us feel fearful, to worry about tomorrow and have guilt about yesterday) the more we are brought into a slower vibration. And because reality is holographic the more we believe something the more we help in creating it.

Information is the key because this physical matrix, this illusionary reality is based on misinformation. You being kept in the dark and in fear (about your body). When a system becomes highly destabilised there are randomn shifts that suddenly self organise into higher complexity.

At the subatomic level reality behaves in accordance with the expectation of the observer. And these particles are simply fluctuations of energy in a void of energy potential. And if you can change the field then you change the behaviour of the atoms.

So feelings we have in our heart are changing the field which in turn changes the atoms so we are literally altering our physical body.

The reality we see is a tiny range of energy within an infinite energy field with infinite frequency ranges

Everywhere we look with the expectation that something will be there, in that act of looking, of observation is the act that creates something for us to see. We are actually building this universe as we go. We are conscious creators and we can create the body we desire, or better still allow the cells to create a body beyond our wildest imaginings.

Mandala colouring takes you into the void and provides a simple constructive device to begin recreating higher frequency versions of yourself including a new improved and incorruptable body if you can hold and maintain that higher vibration through your own Lovingness.

A Final Word

When you realize that there is no more fight, that there is nothing more to battle, that what you saw is all old stuff and it is all over, you will realize that all your thoughts have been but a passing panorama of your human experience. The only thing you have to win over are your own thought patterns.

This is accomplished by a gentle, loving, understanding, and non judgmental attitude to self. Mandalas become a valuable tool in this endeavour. Come to mandalas with an open mind, a playful heart, and you will create miracles.

Your transformation is through the total allowance of the Great Flow to be the background of your entire experiencing. It is when you can trust and allow this Flow to work in your life that Grace enters you. It becomes eternally present in your awareness. In this Grace you are flooded with a Presence that begins to 'take your breathe away'. You breathe more deeply, more consciously and it flows in and through your life, touching everything about you and around you. And the Presence takes you over, you begin to become it and it becomes you.

The knowing of this leads you to let go more because in your life, you begin to see that absolutely everything is taken care of. It all happens so easily so effortlessly. Wellness arrives because there is nothing more to fix, to release, to "work" through. Just a simple choice of experiencing the up and down motion of human experience as an opportunity to test your wings and discover what thoughts you will pay attention to and allow to play in your life. The rest, the majority of the thoughts, you will allow to pass, to fall way without giving them any attention.

You find that you can create by the simplest intention of thought and that you no longer wait for results because you know, without any shadow of doubt, that in the Flow, in this state of Grace, all is most beautifully present even though you do not see it immediately. The mandala experience can make a significant contribution to teaching you these things. And like miracles, sometimes your simple intentions can manifest in almost instantaneous, unexpected, and surprising ways. Life becomes a magnificent dance of allowance in Love.

So in fact there is no more battle for health, no more fatal sickness or loss. There are brief moments of appearing to hold on and then there is Flow.

Allow Grace to enter. Let go and trust yourself, your inner process and the benevolence of all Creation. If nothing else when you enter this mandala activity with openness, Grace will enter and be present and you will know it to be so.

Nicky Hamid

Internet Colouring Pages

Here is a small list of the many free, printable

Mandala coloring pages available on the Internet.

http://mandalaz.free.fr/fr/mandalas_grands.html

http://www.mandalarbre.com/volume_1.htm

http://www.mandalarbre.com/volume_2.htm

http://www.mandalarbre.com/volume_3.htm

http://amind.co.kr/en/?gclid=CNSEuc2ku54CFSUsawod2ia
4lg

http://coloringpagesforkids.info/free-kaleidoscope-
coloring-pages/

http://www.hellokids.com/c_3790/coloring/mandalas-
gallery-coloring-pages/mandala-coloring-pages-
advanced-level/oriental-mandala-coloring-page

http://coloringpages.nick-magic.com/mandalas.html

http://www.livingwordsofwisdom.com/mandala-coloring-
pages.html

Crop Circle Drawings by Zef Damen

http://www.zefdamen.nl/CropCircles/en/Crop_circles_en.h
tm

Contact Information

If this book has resonated with you please consider giving feedback and a rating to Amazon. Even a couple of lines would be appreciated.

I write on similar topics almost every day on Facebook. Please consider becoming a subscriber where you can share with a family of others around the world. You would be most welcome.

Facebook: www.facebook.com/nicky.hamid.5

Website: www.quantumselfhealing.net

A PDF file is available containing **100 mandalas** on this website for a small charge.

Books: All You Can Be: Empowering Awakening Angels. www.angelsawakening.net/book.php

All You Can Be describes how we are experiencing this deep rooted revolution in the very nature of ourselves and our reality. It outlines the widespread symptoms of this transformation and the extraordinary new potential for growth in awareness and creative expression. It traces an expanded view of our origin and nature and points to the new base of knowledge and empowerment being firmly anchored in an intuitive and heartfelt guidance system.
Email: nickyhamid@gmail.com Please let me know if you have any questions or comments.

About the Author

Growing up in NZ Nicky was inspired by his mother to explore comparative religion at an early age. He completed his Ph.D in psychology in record time and has taught at universities for over thirty years, in psychology, self-awareness, human potential, and the psychology in religion, endeavouring to integrate the rigid confines of the discipline with the teachings of the mystic schools and the path of enlightenment. He has conducted spiritual retreats and self-awareness workshops throughout New Zealand, and in a number of other countries.

He currently maintains a worldwide spiritual mentoring service and continues to speak and conduct workshops.

A Call to Readers

I would very much appreciate any feedback on experiences you have with mandala colouring in order to build a resource that will give others confidence to empower themselves on their own journey.

Please feel free to email me at nickyhamid@gmail.com with any experiences of the activation process you may have mentally, emotionally, or with physical symptoms. Insights, resolutions, or transformations that you feel have been a direct result of your work are welcome.

May your journey be filled with the miracles of welcome and unexpected surprises.

Good Health and Peace

Nicky

Made in the USA
Lexington, KY
28 July 2013